Beat your allergies

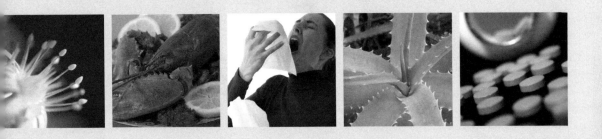

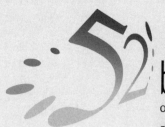

brilliantideas

one good idea can change your life...

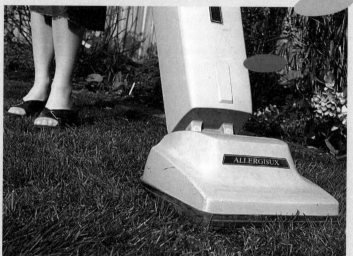

Beat your allergies

Find relief, feel free

Dr Rob Hicks

CAREFUL NOW...

The disclaimers in medical books and on the internet are getting longer. Sometimes these lines of microscopic print take up more space than the content itself. They may even contribute to triggering a person's allergy symptoms, which is not what we want to happen when you read this book. So we're keeping this brief and to the point.

Beat Your Allergies is intended to inform, entertain and provoke the thinking of the reader. It is provided for general information only, and should not be treated as a substitute for the medical advice of your own doctor or other health care professional. Whilst every effort has been made to provide accurate and up-to-date information, medical science is constantly evolving. Neither the author nor the publisher can be held responsible or liable for any loss or claim arising out of the use, or misuse, of the suggestions made in this book. We don't know your specific circumstances and so we're not suggesting any specific course of action for you to follow. It's your health, it's your life and so it makes sense for you to weigh up carefully the choices available and to decide what action, if any, you might take. If in doubt you should always consult your doctor for individualised health and medical advice.

I would like to thank Allergy UK, who provide excellent information about allergies for the general public, for their advice and support. They can be contacted at:
Allergy UK
No. 3 White Oak Square
London Road
Swanley
Kent BR8 7AG
Tel: +44 (0)1322 619898
http://www.allergyuk.org

First published in 2005 by
The Infinite Ideas Company Limited
36 St Giles
Oxford
OX1 3LD
United Kingdom
www.infideas.com

CIP catalogue records for this book are available from the British Library and the US Library of Congress.

ISBN 1-904902-43-X

Brand and product names are trademarks or registered trademarks of their respective owners.

Designed and typeset by Baseline Arts Ltd, Oxford
Printed and bound by TJ International, Cornwall

Brilliant ideas

Brilliant features

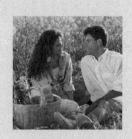

Each chapter of this book is designed to provide you with an inspirational idea that you can read quickly and put into practice straight away.

Throughout you'll find four features that will help you to get right to the heart of the idea:

■ *Here's an idea for you* Give it a go – right here, right now – and get an idea of how well you're doing so far.

■ *Try another idea* If this idea looks like a life-changer then there's no time to lose. *Try another idea* will point you straight to a related tip to expand and enhance the first.

■ *Defining ideas* Words of wisdom from masters and mistresses of the art, plus some interesting hangers-on.

■ *How did it go?* If at first you do succeed try to hide your amazement. If, on the other hand, you don't this is where you'll find a Q and A that highlights common problems and how to get over them.

Introduction

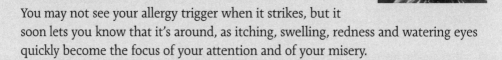

'The fight is won or lost far away from witnesses – behind the lines, in the gym, and out there on the road, long before I dance under those lights.'
MUHAMMAD ALI

You may not see your allergy trigger when it strikes, but it soon lets you know that it's around, as itching, swelling, redness and watering eyes quickly become the focus of your attention and of your misery.

It's now estimated that in the UK approximately one in four people will be affected by an allergy at some time in their life. Over the past fifty years or so the number of people suffering with allergies has increased dramatically and doesn't show any sign of slowing down.

Nobody is sure why allergies are on the increase. Popular beliefs about pollution, poor diets and our lives being over-hygienic are still only theories. Only time and extensive research will provide a clear explanation. Until that wonderful dawning is upon us it's important to do what we can in the battle against our allergies.

Whatever allergy you may have, whether it be hayfever, perennial rhinitis, food allergy, latex allergy, eczema or asthma, if left to its own devices it will interfere with your life in one way or another. Maybe it will be just an occasional nuisance, but it may take over your life, stopping you from doing what you want to do and being who you want to be. And that is why it's important to do whatever you can to avoid becoming a victim of your allergy.

There are lots of simple lifestyle changes that will help you to keep your allergies at bay, which will put you firmly in the driving seat. These lifestyle changes may not work overnight, but given time and your continued efforts they'll help you succeed in achieving your goal.

And that's what this book is all about. It's not about scaring you so near to death that you give up and cocoon yourself away from the world at specific times of the year (or all year round for that matter). It's about the principles of allergy management, and how simple but effective ideas, 52 of them to be precise, can help you to take control of your allergy.

Some of the ideas need you to make a little bit of effort, others need no more than you to be willing to give them a try. Many of them may make you think, 'Surely this can't make a difference?' Once you've tried them, you'll see that they can. Whilst trying the different ideas, you should have fun. None of them are meant to punish you. Putting the ideas into practice will not leave your pockets empty either, but they may leave you with a smile on your face.

'I got the bill for my surgery. Now I know what those doctors were wearing masks for.'
JAMES H. BOREN

Defining idea...

Every day, what you do impacts on your health. It either makes it better or makes it worse. Keeping healthy is actually very simple. Healthy eating, regular exercise, not smoking, not drinking too much alcohol and keeping stress under control are the basics of good health. On paper it's easy, but what is much harder is putting all these principles into practice, and then sticking to them.

This is why making small but effective lifestyle changes works. They are straightforward to do and they slip easily into everyday life, quickly becoming part of your normal daily routine. Before long you'll be reaching for your shades, vacuuming with glee, taking five minutes to relax and doing much, much more without even having to think about it. And as an added bonus, it isn't just your allergies that will benefit – your overall physical and emotional health will improve too.

If you are worried that this is a textbook about allergies, relax. It's not. And before you ask, the only tests will be those you set yourself. This is a book that I hope offers you practical and common-sense advice about how you can keep your allergy under control so that instead of being excluded you'll be able to enjoy life to the full. I have many years of professional experience of allergy, and some personal experience too, and know how having an allergy can interfere with a person's life. I've learned about what works to keep allergies under control and what doesn't, not only from other doctors, but also from my patients, who have been kind enough to share their ideas with me. I've also seen the look of relief and, dare I say, pride on the faces of those who've been able to say 'I don't have any symptoms, I've got my allergy under control' as a result of them putting ideas like these into practice.

I can feel that you're ready to get started. So off you go, and enjoy.

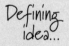
Defining idea...

'The truth of the matter is that you always know the right thing to do. The hard part is doing it.'
GENERAL H. NORMAN SCHWARZKOPF

1

Going into overdrive

You've heard the term allergy because, let's face it, the word is everywhere. But do you know what it really is? Let's scratch the surface and rub away some of the myths.

Never before have so many people suffered at the hands of allergy. Millions around the globe are sniffing, sneezing, wiping and scratching right now.

Think back to a time when you've gone off at the deep end for no real reason. Maybe the bus pulled away just as you reached the stop, or the lift doors closed just before you could wedge your hand in the gap and squeeze yourself inside. Mildly frustrating perhaps, though ultimately harmless – but regardless of this, you still went off on one. Well this is what happens with allergies. Substances such as pollen, mould, animal dander and house dust mite droppings, which under normal circumstances are perfectly harmless, send the immune system into action. Like the way the person who jumped the queue in front of you got you riled, these substances, called allergens, trigger an allergic reaction in the body. Even feeling stressed can trigger allergy symptoms to be set off.

Here's an idea for you...

Next time you find yourself in a situation that might trigger you to overreact – for example, when you can't get a signal on your mobile or the bank's cash machine tells you it's out of service – just take a deep breath in and out whilst counting to ten. Doing this will prevent you from getting yourself wound up and triggering your allergy symptoms.

Each and every one of us has something amazing within us – a heart. But we also have something else that is equally impressive, and that's our immune system. It's what protects us when undesirables get inside us. It protects us from the nasties that may be in the air we breathe, the food we eat and the things we touch. Bacteria and viruses are common invaders that the immune system deals with quite easily when they come our way. Basically the immune system is the body's army, and it's a well-equipped one.

It's also a well-trained one. It's trained to recognise what's on its side, for example the normal cells of the intestines. It's also able to distinguish what's not on its side but is nevertheless safe, like roast chicken, and what's not on its side but is dangerous, such as a *Campylobacter* infection, which causes food poisoning.

Some people are predisposed to developing allergies. When the allergen, or trigger substance, enters the body for the first time specific types of defensive antibodies are produced. The immune system becomes sensitised to these allergens, whether they be pollen, animal dander or specific food types. It's rather like a soldier being taught how to recognise the enemy and having the necessary weapons available to deal with it. You see, these allergens, just like bacteria and viruses, can enter and attack the body in a variety of ways. They may be inhaled into the nose and the lungs, ingested by mouth, or injected or absorbed through the skin. Squads of the body's specific defensive antibodies position themselves in strategic positions around the body. They also attach themselves to mast cells – the storage centre or weapons armoury, which contains stockpiles of the necessary chemicals needed to cause an allergic reaction – and then they just wait for allergens to appear.

To find out about a variety of allergies run along to IDEA 2, All men are not equal.

Try another idea...

Each type of antibody is programmed to recognise a particular allergen, for example pollen. When the allergen enters the body, the specific antibody trained to recognise it captures it and initiates a full-blown attack. It does this by causing the mast cell to release its load of histamine and other chemicals. Some of these substances are responsible for giving the orders, while others are involved in the actual combat and getting the job done. Some of these chemicals call in support from other teams that then make their way to the war zone and join in the battle. It is the effects of these chemicals that produce the symptoms of the allergy attack: in the case of pollen, this includes sneezing, a runny nose and itching eyes.

The problem with allergy is that the allergens, such as pollen, are normally considered harmless. In most people, if these substances enter the body they would cause no symptoms at all. They are innocent bystanders. But in those who have an allergy, wrong information – or bad intelligence, to continue the war analogy – means that the immune system is primed to react when it need not do so. Instead of reading, say, a red cross as a sign of neutrality, it reads it as a series of concentric circles with a bull's-eye in the middle. And what happens is described by the military as friendly fire.

'A little more moderation would be good, my life hasn't exactly been one of moderation.'
DONALD TRUMP

Defining idea...

3

How did it go?

Q   Why do some substances trigger allergies but not others?

A   *It is still not fully understood why some substances trigger allergies in susceptible people whilst other substances do not. It's also not clear why some people develop an allergic reaction after exposure to specific allergens while others don't. There are a handful of theories to explain why someone develops allergies, but the single most important factor that predisposes a person to develop allergic disease is a family history of it.*

Q   Apparently allergies are on the increase. Why is this?

A   *There are many different possibilities to explain why allergies are increasing, but the precise answer still eludes us. Most people believe that modern Western living plays a large part, since in rural areas of Africa and Asia allergy does not appear to exist. Some allergy may be increasing in line with increasing exposure to house dust mites, because our modern, carpeted, draught-free and warm homes allow them to breed faster than you could say 'Oi! Stop that!' One popular theory is the hygiene hypothesis. We are all too clean, and so are our homes. Consequently a lack of exposure to harmless bacteria means that the immune system does not get the appropriate training and programming it needs in early childhood. Passive smoking may also play a part in the development of allergies, as may a lack of fruit and vegetables in the diet. Time will hopefully provide more answers, but at the moment although we have theories we still have many questions.*

2

All men are not equal

Neither are all allergies equal, or indeed the same. Allergies come in different forms, so here's a quick guide to the common culprits.

Allergies come in all shapes and sizes, and affect people in different ways. Some are just a nuisance, others make life a misery, whilst a few threaten life itself.

Hayfever is probably the most well known allergy, and can make having fun in spring and summer impossible for many sufferers. Stories of how a school examination performance was hindered because of hayfever are true. If streaming eyes mean you can't see the examination paper clearly, which is soaked through anyway from your dripping nose and continual sneezing, and your blocked nose means your mate has no idea what you're saying when you ask to see his answers, how can you expect to do well? And it's not only the eyes and nose that pollen irritates, it can cause the roof of the mouth and the ears to itch as well.

If you think hayfever, or seasonal rhinitis, is bad, spare a thought for those with *perennial* allergic rhinitis, who basically get the symptoms of hayfever all year round.

Here's an idea for you...

Each morning, before you bathe or shower, let the hot water run for a while as you inhale the steam. Once you've showered or bathed, moisturise your whole body. Finally, drink a glass of fresh water and eat breakfast. By doing this you'll start your day with a clear nose, soft skin, and a hydrated and fuelled body, giving yourself the best chance of keeping allergy symptoms at bay.

They're the people in your office who appear to always have a cold. It's usually the dung of the house dust mite that's been getting up their nose whilst their continual sniffing has been getting up yours.

Eczema is also known as dermatitis, which just means inflammation of the skin. The word eczema comes from the Greek language and means 'to boil over' or 'to erupt', which describes perfectly what happens when the skin becomes dry, itchy, red, inflamed and weepy. The commonest type occurs in childhood and is called atopic eczema (atopic meaning that the person is allergic, or allergy-prone). Another type of eczema, more often found in adults, is contact eczema. Although, strictly speaking, it's a sensitivity rather than an allergy, those who suffer from it find that contact with a substance triggers their skin to become red, inflamed and itchy. The usual culprits are metals, such as nickel, and substances in perfumes and household cleaning products.

Coughing, wheezing and shortness of breath are all typical of asthma. With asthma, the airways become narrow as a result of inflammation, excessive mucus and airway muscle contraction, and this, in turn, obstructs the airflow within the lungs. Remember when, as a kid, you'd wrestle with your older brother, sister or classmate and they'd sit on your chest? Well that sort of constriction is how it feels for someone when they are having an asthma attack. In fact, it can feel like all three are sitting on you at the same time!

Admiring the wild flowers and picking blackberries from the hedgerows in the countryside is idyllic until ouch, you've brushed against nettles and been stung. Nettle rash or hives (or urticaria, to give it its medical name) causes itchy, raised white bumps

You've had some fun trying one idea – now it's time to get serious. Take a look at IDEA 19, *Anaphylaxis*, to learn what to do in this medical emergency.

Try another idea...

surrounded by red, swollen inflammation on the skin where histamine in the liquid from the nettle itself has been injected into the skin and where the body has reacted by releasing its own histamine too. This same reaction on the skin can also occur as a result of other triggers, such as in food or drug allergy reactions.

For some people mild reactions to food, such as tingling of the lips, may be the only effect of food allergy. However, for others just brief contact with the offending substance can be enough to provoke swelling of the face, lips, tongue and throat. They may look like a cartoon character, but it's not funny. Life-threatening anaphylaxis may also occur at the same time.

And this is what everybody fears – anaphylaxis. The most severe form of allergic reaction, it's a medical emergency as it can be fatal. On the shortlist of triggers are food, insect stings and bites, medications, vaccines and latex. If someone develops nettle rash, swollen skin, describes a sense of impending doom, is hoarse, light-headed, has difficulty breathing or chest tightness, it's important to think anaphylaxis and get medical help immediately.

'My theory is that if you look confident you can pull off anything – even if you have no clue what you are doing.'
JESSICA ALBA, American actress.

Defining idea...

7

Q   Is it possible to have more than one type of allergy?

A   *Yes, it is. If people who are atopic (that is, allergy-prone) have one allergy, such as hayfever, then they are far more likely to have other allergies, such as eczema and asthma. This doesn't mean that they are definitely going to get more than one allergy; it simply means that they have an underlying tendency to allergy that may become activated.*

Q   My brother has various allergies and there is a history of allergies in other members of my family, but I don't seem to be allergic to anything. Is it possible that I will not develop allergies or am I an allergy-ticking time bomb?

A   *It sounds as if your family is atopic and it is likely that you carry the genes for allergy, since they are likely to have been passed to you from your parents. However, it is also possible that you will never develop allergies. Current understanding is that our genes predict whether we may develop an allergy, and then environmental stimuli – diet, hygiene (where less appears to be better!), house design for example – determine whether allergic conditions develop or not. Since it's now believed that how allergy-prone people are probably depends upon the number of different allergy-influencing genes they inherit, it is possible for one sibling to inherit lots, giving them a strong tendency towards developing allergies, whilst another sibling inherits fewer, meaning they have a weaker tendency to develop allergy.*

3

Intolerable cruelty

Now don't take this personally but, although you may think you have an allergy, in reality you may just be intolerant. Take a bite of this to see why allergies get upset by intolerance.

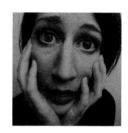

This behaviour will not be tolerated. Do you understand me? Now, go to your room until you can settle down and behave sensibly.

You must have been on the receiving end of this; we all have. The room was invariably our bedroom, which nowadays for children is more of a treat than a punishment, since many have their own TV, computer and even phone in there. And presumably this is why parents are never sent to their room: they'd welcome the chance to grab some uninterrupted sleep. With food intolerance, however, having to go to, and remain in, the room – often the bathroom – is a real punishment for those who suffer.

Food intolerance can be responsible for an enormous variety of symptoms, the more common ones including headache, diarrhoea, bloating, nausea, aching muscles and joints, and fatigue. It often causes a general feeling of ill-health that is difficult to pinpoint. Whereas food allergy symptoms are usually sudden and

Here's an idea for you...

If you suffer with symptoms that you think may be caused by your being intolerant to certain foods, try keeping a food and symptoms diary for a couple of weeks. Write down all the food you eat and the symptoms you experience, and when you eat or experience them. This will help you to identify possible food triggers for your symptoms and will help your doctor to make a diagnosis too.

sometimes potentially fatal, the symptoms of food intolerance tend to be more gradual and life-irritating rather than life-threatening. For example, you may eat a sandwich at lunchtime then later in the afternoon feel uncomfortable, perhaps bloated, or are stuck in the toilet, diarrhoea dictating your every movement.

Food intolerance has the potential to upset more than the just the person who suffers with it too. This is because the current popular trend is to put every unexplained medical complaint down to an 'allergy'. For some reason, allergies are seen as fashionable. For example, I know one parent who was furious to be told that her six-year old didn't have an allergy, but simply had food intolerance. 'All her friends have got allergies! How's she going to feel being the only one without one?' The parent should have been relieved. Of course, it's unlikely that all her daughter's friends have allergies. Some may have had food intolerances with the balance probably being just fads and fancies.

Food allergies and food intolerance are fundamentally different. Food allergy results from the immune system reacting inappropriately to harmless substances within the food. In contrast, food intolerance does not involve the immune system but occurs in response to substances in food that may be toxic to some individuals. Difficulties arise because medical understanding of food intolerance is in its infancy;

the media likes to promote allergy as being responsible for all our ills, whether they be headaches, tiredness, inadequate sexual performance or rising interest rates; and charlatans – those people who offer inaccurate, unscientific and unproven allergy tests and who eagerly replace the holes they've created in your diet and your wallet with various allergy-conquering supplements – have jumped on the opportunity to make a quick buck by preying on the vulnerable intolerants. However, tests that identify specific antibodies (IgG antibodies) to food are now available and in clinical research have shown great promise in helping to accurately identify which foods someone may be intolerant to.

So you can see why there's growing intolerance. Doctors are irritated by those who don't have an allergy complaining about their 'allergy', those with allergies feel that their condition is being undervalued, and those with food intolerance feel frustrated because currently medical science can't provide a satisfactory explanation for their very real problem even though it's got a good idea about what to do about it. So let's try and be more tolerant to those around us and keep peace and harmony in the world both outside and inside us.

Now you've got a handle on intolerance, take a nibble of IDEA 43, *Should it stay or should it go?*, to see how elimination can help to make things more tolerable.

Try another idea...

'Anger and intolerance are the twin enemies of correct understanding.'
MAHATMA GANDHI

Defining idea...

How did
it go?

Q   My doctor said that I have idiopathic food intolerance. What is this?

A   *Basically it means that there is no apparent mechanism for your food intolerance, and that the doctor doesn't know why you react in the way you do. It's not because your doctor is thick, it's because the reason just isn't known yet. Many people have idiopathic food intolerance, and in time hopefully science will identify more precisely why such intolerance occurs. Some people do know what causes their food intolerance. Some, for example, have metabolic abnormalities, the most common being a lactase enzyme deficiency that causes lactose intolerance.*

Q   I think I have food intolerance. How can I treat it?

A   *To begin with, it's important to establish that your symptoms are being caused by a food or foods, because if they're not, then treating them as food intolerance is unlikely to help. Keeping a food diary and then using an appropriate elimination diet should help to uncover the culprit or culprits. Then the best way to treat the problem is simply not to eat the foods you've identified as being triggers for your symptoms.*

Q   I don't have food allergy or food intolerance, so why should I care what it is or worry about what I eat?

A   *You probably know someone with a food allergy or food intolerance, so having some understanding will help you to help and tolerate them. Diet is important for good health, so try focusing on your diet to make sure that you eat the recommended five portions of fruit and vegetables a day, and that you reduce your consumption of fat (particularly saturated fat) and sugary foods.*

4

Sticking up your nose

A magnet for fingers, the nose is also the entry point for many of the allergy troublemakers. Fool them into thinking they'll have a smooth passage and with this idea you'll soon have them trapped.

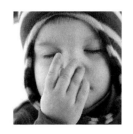

If we were not supposed to put our fingers up our nose, then why do they fit so well? That's most people's excuse, but feel free to pick your own.

Of course, it's not only fingers that find their way into the nose. Most talked about, I suppose, is the white powder given celebrity by pop stars and city bankers. Small children love to stick things like sweetcorn, plastic beads and toy soldiers up their noses – basically anything they can get their hands on. But there are things that can legitimately be guided into the dark recesses of the nasal passages. Medicinal creams and microscopic droplets of liquid, for instance. Another favourite that can certainly help those with nasal allergies is, believe it or not, petroleum jelly.

It was Robert Augustus Cheesebrough, a chemist in Brooklyn, who noticed that oil workers would slap the colourless film called 'rod wax', which collected around the

You know it's in your medicine cabinet somewhere, so go and get the petroleum jelly. Gently smear some around the inside of your nose. By doing this before you go out each day you will help your nose to filter out the irritants, and not only will you suffer fewer nasal allergy problems, you may also find yourself breathing more freely too.

pump rods on the oil wells, on a cut instead of a bandage. This 'rod wax' not only stayed on the skin and stopped the bleeding, it seemed to help cure the wound too. He developed a clean form of it and gave it the name 'petroleum jelly'. The story has it that he made so much of the stuff that he struggled to find places to keep it, and so had to use his wife's flower vases to store it. Since new oil-based products of the time ended in 'ine', he added this to the word 'vase' and so was born the name we know today– 'Vaseline Petroleum Jelly'.

Petroleum jelly may no longer be used in the immediate treatment of burns, but it still has a number of health uses. Who amongst us hasn't had some smeared on our lips to protect them from the chaffing cold winds? It can protect and moisturise dry skin, and can bring relief to skin irritation. Shoved into the nose, it can help control allergies too.

Although often the source of humour, let's give credit where credit is due: the nose is an amazing piece of kit. Stuck on the middle of the face, it's one of the first things we notice when we meet people. Whether you've a small or large, perfectly symmetrical or slightly off-centre scenter, it adds a great deal of character and enables us to be recognised, and to recognise others. In fact, the nose attracts a great deal of attention, not least that of plastic surgeons, emphasised by the fact that the nose job continues to be one of the most popular cosmetic operations. Of course, the nose has other, more responsible, functions to fulfil than merely looking distinctive. It's our own unique air-conditioner, moistening and warming up cold air before it travels to the lungs. It's also a fantastic filtration system. The fine hairs that line the inside of the nose filter out and trap any undesirable particles that are hitching a ride in the air. As part of this clean-up process, the nose makes sticky mucus to help with the same job.

And this is where petroleum jelly comes into it's own. Not only is a light smearing around the inside of the nostrils soothing to dry, cracked skin – which, let's face it, soon manifests when the nose is running and in need of a wipe every few minutes – it also helps to trap the little blighters such as pollen grains before they can get further in and start irritating.

And if you think of your finger as a rod, smearing petroleum jelly around it and rubbing it around the inside of your nose is simply using the jelly in the same way as it was first discovered by those 19th-century oil workers.

If you enjoyed this idea, take a sip of IDEA 17, *Water, water everywhere*, to find out how water can actually be of help if you have allergies.

Try another idea...

'The sense of humor is the oil of life's engine.'
GEORGE S. MERRIAM, American publisher

Defining idea...

15

How did it go?

Q   Does the jelly have to go all the way inside the nose?

A   *No. Just a little bit inside the opening will do. If you try to put it too far inside then you may cause some irritation as you try and sweep your finger full circle around the nostril. Also, remember that the purpose of the jelly is to trap particles before they get too far inside the nose, so it needs to be near the outside. Putting the jelly too far inside may actually gum up the fine hairs preventing them from working properly and giving irritant invaders an easy passage.*

Q   How often should it be replaced?

A   *If you have hayfever, try applying some five or ten minutes before you go outside. During the day you may well need to wipe or blow your nose, in which case you'll need to reapply some jelly each time. It's not a bad idea to gently wipe away the jelly every few hours anyway, to remove anything that it has caught and to apply some more. On high pollen count days you may need to reapply it more frequently.*

Q   Do you have to have hayfever to try this?

A   *Not at all. You can try it to help with any allergy where irritants get in through the nose. For example, if you have perennial allergic rhinitis (basically, this is hayfever symptoms all year round), you can try the petroleum jelly idea, but you have to do it when you are indoors too since the commonest irritant, or allergen, is the dung of the house dust mite.*

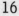

Thanks for buying one of our books! If you'd like to be placed on our mailing list to receive more information on forthcoming releases in the **52 Brilliant Ideas** series just send an e-mail to *info@infideas.com* with your name and address or simply fill in the details below and pop this card in the post. No postage is needed. We promise we won't do silly things like bombard you with lots of junk mail, nor would we even consider letting third parties look at your details. Ever.

Name:...

Address:...

....

e-mail:...

Which book did you purchase?...................................

....

Tell us what you thought of this book and our series; check out the 'Brilliant Communication' bit on the other side of this card.

I am interested in the following subjects:

☐ Health & relationships
☐ Lifestyle & leisure
☐ Arts, literature and music

☐ Careers, finance & personal development
☐ Sports, hobbies & games
☐ Actually, I'd be quite interested in:...

And just to say thanks, every month we'll pick 3 random names from a hat (ok, it may be some other cylindrical device) and send a complimentary book from the series. It could be you. So please tell us what book you'd like:...(check out www.52brilliantideas.com for a full list of our titles, or if you prefer we can choose one for you based on your subject interest).

You can change your life with brilliant ideas.

We're passionate about the effect our books have and we have designed them so that they can become an inspiring part of your daily routine. Our books help people to grow, giving them the confidence to believe in themselves and to transform their lives. Every day, around the world, people are regaining control of their lives with our brilliant ideas.

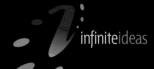
infiniteideas

www.52brilliantideas.com

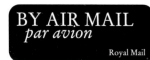
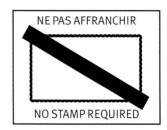
Brilliant Communication

- If you enjoyed this book and find yourself cuddling it at night, please tell us. If you think this book isn't fit to use as kindling, please let us know. We value your thoughts and need your honest feedback. We know if we listen to you we'll get it right. Why not send us an e-mail at *listeners@infideas.com*.

- Do you have a brilliant idea of your own that our author has missed? E-mail us at *yourauthor missedatrick@infideas.com* and if it makes it into print in a future edition or appears on our web site we'll send you four books of your choice OR the cash equivalent. You'll be fully credited (if you want) so that everyone knows you've had a brilliant idea.

- Finally, if you've enjoyed one of our books why not become an **Infinite Ideas Ambassador**. Simply e-mail ten of your friends enlightening them about the virtues of the **52 Brilliant Ideas** series and dishing out our web address: www.52brilliantideas.com. Make sure you copy us in at *ambassador@infideas.com*. We promise we won't contact them unless they contact us, but we'll send you a free book of your choice for every ten friends you email. Help spread the word!

5

It's a wrap

We all know that sunglasses protect the eyes from the sun and make us look cool, but there's more to them than that. Check out the shades, as if you needed an excuse, and see what they can do for allergies.

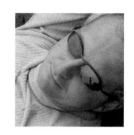

You may not be a Hollywood star, but it doesn't matter. You have every right to don a pair of cool shades too.

In days gone by it was mostly the rich and famous who wore shades. Their eyewear symbolised success and wealth. Despite them claiming that they kept their eyes covered to avoid the public eye – nowadays it would be to avoid the retina-burning paparazzi flashguns – we all know that the opposite was true. Wearing shades was a cry for attention, a way to stand out in a crowd. Basically their sunglasses were saying, 'look at me, I'm famous'. (Now talking sunglasses – that's cool!) After all, who else would wear dark shades at night?

But could there be another reason for them to be wearing shades? Perhaps we shouldn't be so quick to judge. Amongst the many advantages these idols of the movie and pop world have access to, such as the limousines, private jets, designer

Here's an idea for you...

Have a look in your drawers and cupboards for any pair of shades. Now wear them and see how much easier your eyes feel for doing so. Wraparound shades are great for keeping pollen out of your eyes, and those with foam seals are even better. So not only will you look good, you'll feel good too.

clothes and more homes than there are days in the week, they also use the best health specialists. Maybe they all suffer with allergies and their health gurus have suggested that they wear shades to protect their eyes.

Just like UV rays can creep in around the sides of some shades and find their way into the eye, so can pollen. If it can get in, it can cause harm. It's a stealth attack, because you won't know that pollen has been there until it's done the damage and you want to scratch your eyes out of their sockets to relieve the itching, watering and pain. You'll do this even though you know that, once you've enjoyed the brief interlude of ecstasy that the rubbing brings, the problem will return immediately and with a vengeance.

Let's be honest, many stars have made a particular style of sunglasses their trademark. Bono of U2, for example. Now manufacturers can't wait to get their frames onto the faces of the world's celebrities. I hold my hands up: when the movie *Top Gun* was released, I saved my pennies for a pair of Ray Ban Aviators, just like every would-be Maverick in town. Don't tell me you didn't fancy a pair of shades to make you look like one of the Men in Black or one of the stars of *The Matrix*. Well, here's your justification.

Basically you need to protect and secure your eyes. On any day when troublesome pollen is likely to be around, especially windy days when it's being blown all over the place, wearing a pair of shades is a good idea. And this is what shades are also designed to do: protect the eyes – from damaging UV light, and from dust, flies, grit, pollen or anything else that cares to come your way.

OK, cut. It's a wrap! Time for you to try IDEA 22, *Risky business*, now that you've sorted your shades and are looking cool.

Try another idea...

Manufacturers have recognised this and have designed shades to fulfil people's specific needs. Take cycling, for example. Downhill cycling or cycling into a headwind can give the eyes a rather unpleasant bashing, to put it mildly. You can close your mouth to keep unwanted bug entry to a minimum, but you can't very well shut your eyes. Wraparound shades offer protection and also style, which to many is just as important. Even the media celebrity bug-eye shades can help so long as you don't mind looking like a sci-fi B-movie extra.

Some manufacturers have taken technology a step further and designed sunglasses that offer the eyes complete protection by incorporating orbital foam seals. Just as swimming goggles prevent water from entering the eyes, so shades with orbital foam seals protect the eyes from wind-borne dust and pollen. Yes, it may be nice to have certain exotic bodies in your line of vision, but you don't want them getting into your eyes and triggering the maddening symptoms of hayfever or any other eye irritation for that matter, now do you?

'I base my fashion taste on what doesn't itch.'
GILDA RADNER, American actress and comedian

Defining idea...

19

How did it go?

Q **I feel a little self-conscious wearing shades. Particularly if not many other people are. Can't I pass on this one?**

A *Think about it this way. More and more people are wearing shades, and more of the time. It has become a popular fashion statement. Anyway, you'll look worse and feel more self-conscious if people are staring at your bloodshot, watering and swollen eyes, won't you? So, given that people will look at you anyway, you might as well be comfortable while they do it!*

Q **It's difficult gardening with shades on – it makes it too dark to see clearly. Any advice for me as a hayfever sufferer?**

A *The simple solution is to let someone else do the gardening for you during your hayfever season. OK, may not be possible, and you don't want to lose this pleasure. So try wearing swimming goggles. They're inexpensive, and will offer your eyes some protection from pollen or anything that wings its way towards your eyes whilst you're strimming the edges. Go for non-tinted ones so you'll be able to see clearly, though remember that these will probably not offer you UV protection. And don't be embarrassed – the only people who are likely to see you are nosy neighbours, and they'll probably take one look and then try to avoid you.*

Q **I've been wearing wraparound glasses but my eyes still get irritated sometimes. What should I do?**

A *It may be worth you trying a pair with foam seals. However, these can be expensive, so before splashing out some, try washing your sunglasses after use, as pollen can stick to them and then find its way into your eyes.*

6

And so to bed

The bedroom is for relaxation, sleep and sex, so here's how to keep those sniffles and nasal obstructions at bay.

We spend about a third of our lives asleep. Some of this time will be on buses, trains or planes, and a fair amount will be in front of the telly. But most will be in bed.

One of the growing problems of modern-day living is poor sleep. Environmental noise and stress are common causes. The fact that many bedrooms now double as a TV viewing room or office doesn't help either.

But there's another reason why our bed in particular may be keeping us awake instead of surrounding us with sleep, apart from it being old and lumpy. It's because many beds are home (or, to be more precise, toilet) to the house dust mite. And if you are allergic to its droppings, as many people are, the refreshing sleep you crave may not come your way. So you need to reduce your exposure to it.

The house dust mite lives in everyone's home. It likes to feed off the dead skin cells that we humans shed continually. 'Mmmmm', it says as it gobbles them up. 'Ah,

Here's an idea for you...

Try using mite-proof mattress, pillow and duvet covers. Make sure that the pores of the covers are less than 1 micron across, ideally less than 0.5 microns, since house dust mite droppings can be as small as this. This should reduce your exposure to the allergens and you should wake up feeling more refreshed after a good night's sleep.

that's better', it sighs as it evacuates what's not wanted. Its dung is a major source of allergic reactions, and the place where it lies in wait for you is your bedroom. House dust mites and their excreta are present elsewhere around the house too, but the major exposure zone is your bed.

Remember those black and white comedy movies where the characters would walk into a dusty old house and the moment they sat down dust would erupt from the furniture and cover them? Well that's what happens when you fluff up cushions, your head hits the pillow or you bounce around on the mattress. Look at sunlight streaming through the bedroom window. Nice, isn't it? But look at all the particles in the air when you thump the pillow. That's millions of dung particles, and if they can get into the air, then they can get into you too. Think about how many times you move in your bed – when you're asleep as well as at other, more energetic, times. Each time you'll be giving yourself a dose of allergen.

It's impossible to keep your bedroom totally clear of house dust mites; they're a fact of life. But one way you can reduce the problems they cause is by using mite-proof allergy reducing covers for mattresses, duvets and pillows. In an ideal world, it's best to put the covers on a brand new mattress, duvet and pillows, which should be mite-free, so that the mites are prevented from getting inside. If this isn't possible, then putting covers on old mattresses and bedding will at least keep the mites inside and stop them getting out and making a nuisance of themselves.

If learning that you've been sleeping on a bed of dung came as a surprise, take a sniff at **IDEA 7, *Household waste*,** and be prepared to be shocked.

Try another idea...

The other guilty party that introduces allergens into the bedroom are pets that spend any time there. Cats are the most common culprits, but dogs, too, can leave their allergen-coated hairs everywhere. Now although the obvious solution would be to lose the pet, this isn't always easy to do. Having your kids wailing through the night as they miss little Tiddles is not going to cure your sleeplessness. So, as an alternative, begin by keeping the pets out of the bedroom at all times. This is necessary as the allergen from pets can remain airborne for hours. It then settles onto soft furnishings, floors and carpets. If you are sensitive to your pet and don't want to break up a happy home, then it makes sense to only allow your pet into those areas of your home where the flooring can be easily cleaned.

Even Teddy may be responsible, or whatever your favoured cuddly toy is, since house dust mites live in these too. But, like pets, this doesn't mean he has to be kicked out – just don't let him have the run of the whole house.

So now you know why, just a few moments after your head hits the pillow, your nose may start feeling stuffy.

'A good laugh and a long sleep are the best cures in the doctor's book.'
IRISH PROVERB

Defining idea...

How did
it go?

Q **I only replaced my bedding a few months ago. I don't want to have to buy more. What can I do?**

A *You can still use mite-proof covers, but try and kill the mites first. Dry-clean the duvet and pillows or, if possible, wash them at 60°C, then put the anti-mite covers on. Washing at a temperature above 55°C kills the mites and removes the dung. It's also possible to have a mattress professionally heat-treated to kill mites that are inside it.*

Q **What should I do with my cuddly toys?**

A *Large families of cuddly toys, which usually live in bedrooms, will be home to millions of house dust mites, so keep the number you have in the bedroom to a minimum. Putting them in a plastic bag in the freezer for 24 hours will kill mites. If the toys are washable, wash them at 60°C afterwards. You can also try putting duvets and pillows in plastic bags and putting them in the freezer for 24 hours at least once a month.*

Q **It didn't do the trick for me. Any suggestions?**

A *Try reducing the concentration of mites and dung in the rest of the bedroom by keeping as few soft furnishings in your bedroom as possible, wet-dusting the bedroom furniture and vacuuming the bedroom floor regularly. Using a vacuum cleaner with a good filter will stop the mites and other small particles being recycled through the cleaner's exhaust. Vacuum the mattress once a week and keep your bedroom well ventilated.*

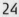

7

Household waste

The toilet isn't the only place where waste needs to be removed. Other rooms are piled up with dung that may be blocking up your systems.

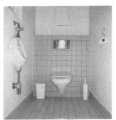

It's everywhere around your home, collecting on everything. It drives mothers to distraction and keeps cleaning product manufacturers rich. The perennial household nightmare — dust.

For some, dusting is an obsession. 'I've just got to give the place a once over because we're expecting visitors', your mother would say. But she's fighting a losing battle, because it's impossible to keep your home completely clear of dust. It comes from the millions of dead skin cells that we shed every day. In addition, the tiny arachnid that is a permanent resident in every home, the house dust mite, feeds on these dead skin cells and forms part of the dust we see around the house.

Here's an idea for you... **When you must do the cleaning or change the bedding yourself, wear a dust mask. You can get one from your local hardware store. It needs to be able to filter out the tiny dung particles, so ideally the pores should be less than 0.5 microns across.**

If you can't rid the family home of this unwelcome occupant, and you're not keen to give yourself a Hannibal Lector-style skin peel to cut off its food supply, is there any hope? Yes, so don't dispair. You may not be able to eradicate it completely, but you can reduce its numbers – and in war, which is what it may feel like, this can make all the difference. If you can reduce the concentration of mites and their dung, and make the environment less homely for them to reinvade, half the battle is won.

The excretion from the mites dries out and can be launched into the air whenever anyone walks over a rug, sits down on a chair or shakes the bedclothes. For those allergic to it, this triggers symptoms that may include a runny nose, itching, sneezing, watering eyes, difficulty in breathing or eczema. Even for those who don't suffer from allergies, entering a dusty room, say the attic, and opening a bag or box that last saw the light of day when telephones were made of Bakelite is enough to send you into paroxysms of coughing and spluttering as the dust hits you. So it is when the irritating house dust mite dung gets into the eyes, nose and mouth of someone who is allergic to it.

The irony is that if we left the dust alone, then yes, it would pile up, but the house dust mite and its dung would probably do us less harm. You see, it's too heavy to float in the air without any help. So when we dust, fluff up pillows and cushions, settle down on the sofa or roll over in bed, we send it flying.

OK, we can't get rid of them completely, so how can we keep down the numbers? House dust mites prefer a humid environment, so having some windows open will reduce their numbers through ventilation and by keeping the air dry. Dehumidifiers can help here too. Mites like soft furnishings, so choosing wood, vinyl or leather-covered furniture where possible means there are fewer places for the mites to live. Keeping dust traps like teddy bears, cushions, dried flowers, bric-a-brac and toys to a minimum helps. If you just can't be without these things, then try and keep them in one room only, a room you don't often use.

It's all very well trying to remove the house dust mite from your home, but what if the family pet's at the root of your problem? Go for a walk to IDEA 8, *Preserving pets*, to see how your pooch may not need to be given the push.

Try another idea...

Wash and vacuum curtains regularly, and think about using lightweight materials for curtains as these tend to collect less dust. When you dust, a damp duster is much more effective than a dry one. Be tidy and always put all clothes away in wardrobes. Where possible, keep your hands off dusty objects. And grandma was right, hanging bedding out to dry outside is a good idea, since sunlight destroys the house dust mite and thoroughly dries bedding, which is essential if mites are not to flourish.

Of course, the perfect solution is to let someone else do the cleaning and housework. This isn't just a good excuse not to do any housework; if you're allergic this means you'll be out of the line of fire when the vacuum cleaner's fan hits the s**t.

'When things don't work well in the bedroom, they don't work well in the living room either.'
WILLIAM H. MASTERS, co-director, Masters & Johnson Institute

Defining idea...

27

How did it go?

Q   Would a cycle mask be any help?

A   *Yes. When you're likely to be exposed to substances that you react to, for example when cleaning your house, wearing a mask is a good idea. Cycle masks are great, and many combine a carbon filter together with a dust filter and so are helpful for those who are sensitive to both indoor and outdoor irritants.*

Q   What's the best advice with regards to vacuuming?

A   *The gold standard is to vacuum daily, but hey, who's got the time? Instead, vacuum as often as is practical, paying particular attention to the bedroom carpet and under your bed. Wear a mask and use a vacuum cleaner with a no-bag vortex and an allergen filter so there's less chance of mites and dung being sprayed into the air. If your skin is what gets irritated, then cover up with clothing to reduce the risk of contact. I know, vacuuming with clothes on sounds pretty radical, but give it a go!*

Q   What are the best floor covers?

A   *There's no easy answer to this, it's about pros and cons. Carpets collect more dust, house dust mites and dung, but they tend to trap them, whereas vinyl and wood floors tend to hoard less dust, mites and dung but allow them to be more easily launched into the air. If you're thinking about removing your carpets, start in the bedroom, since this is the epicentre for house dust mites anyway. Losing the bathroom carpet is also a good idea since it's one of the most humid rooms in the house, so makes a great breeding place. Then see how you get on.*

8

Preserving pets

They bring love, affection and happiness into a home, but for those with allergies giving pets the push may seem like the only solution.

But just as there's more than one way to skin the proverbial cat, there's more than one way to remain at one with your pussy, and with your other pets too.

Not long ago, good friends of mine decided the time had come to allow their children to have pets and home came two wonderful kittens. It was family bliss personified. Well, it was until a few days later, when mum started wheezing. But the cats are still with them, and there's been no more wheezing either. So how did they do it?

Despite popular myth, cat or dog fur is not actually the problem. Even if you were allergic to your pet and took it to the barber for a number one haircut, you'd still find yourself with watery red eyes and coughing. Not because the sight of your best ex-furry friend would reduce you to tears, but because it's actually glands in the animal's skin that secrete allergy-triggering proteins, or allergens, which linger in

Here's an idea for you...

Wash your cat or dog once or twice a week with a regular pet shampoo or water. This will reduce the allergen on the pet and in the air. If even the hint of running water provokes a cat or dogfight, try just wiping her fur each day with a damp cloth.

the animal's fur and float easily into the air. These allergens can be present in the animal's saliva and urine too, and may become airborne when the saliva dries on the fur. So, apart from producing the world's first short-haired Afghan, your trip to the barber's would have achieved nothing. So scalping it isn't the solution. Taxidermy might reduce the number of allergens, though it's a bit extreme, and I've yet to see a stuffed animal obey a command.

The problem with these allergens is that they're not only invisible to the naked eye, they're also lightweight. Just walking through your house is enough to waft them into the air, and what happens next is all too predictable. You inhale these proteins and your trouble starts all over again.

In theory, the answer is simple: reduce your exposure to the allergens. The obvious and, indeed, the best solution, therefore, is to find your loved one a new home. No cat, no exposure. Simple. But don't be tempted to re-home them with friends or relatives, unless, of course, you're looking for an excuse not to see them. 'I'd love to come visit, really I would, but you know what happens.' But understandably you want the best of both worlds, and that means keeping your pet and keeping your allergy at bay.

To begin with, as far as indoor allergy management is concerned, increased ventilation equals decreased allergen, so open a window from time to time.

Nowadays HEPA (that's High-Efficiency Particulate Air, if you're interested) air cleaners and HEPA filters in vacuum cleaners can also help remove allergen from indoor surroundings. When animals give themselves a good licking, or rather a wash, they produce lots of allergen that finds its way into the air, so putting them outdoors to do this can help. This can also avoid those embarrassing moments when your pet insists on a quick genital scrub as your guests are sitting down to their canapés!

Usually it's a compromise between symptom control and cuddling when pets are concerned, so have a look at IDEA 13, *Ah, what a relief*, to see what you can do if a cuddle leaves your eyes and nose streaming.

Try another idea...

In fact, the pet should ideally be kept outdoors in a comfortable and safe environment if you really want to reduce allergen levels indoors, but hey, why do we have pets in the first place? Instead, make some areas of your home off-limits to your pets. The bedroom should without doubt be a no-go area. If you want your pet to follow you wherever you go, then soft furnishings and fitted carpets may need to be shown the door and materials that can be easily wiped clean, such as vinyl, leather and wood, welcomed instead. There's no escaping the need to clean frequently and thoroughly to remove dust and animal dander, and this should include pet beds and blankets too, where allergens are just waiting to take off and irritate you.

'Happiness is having a scratch for every itch.'
OGDEN NASH, American writer and poet

Defining idea...

How did it go?

Q   What's best if you have allergies, a cat or a dog?

A   *All cats and dogs have the potential to cause allergy – even hairless breeds. In general, dog sensitivity occurs less often in allergic people, although some people are more sensitive to dogs than cats. Some even find that a particular cat or dog may cause them more irritation than another of the same breed. Usually the final decision comes down to individual preference.*

Q   I've heard about special anti-allergy shampoos. Do they work?

A   *At the time of writing, the majority view amongst allergy experts is that shampoos marketed for animal allergy are no better than conventional pet shampoos. However, I've spoken with people who are convinced that an anti-allergy shampoo allowed them to live in harmony with their pet. It may be worth trying one, but consult with your vet beforehand as you don't want to harm your pet. Remember, to gain benefit from washing your pet you have to do it regularly, not once in a blue moon.*

Q   Unfortunately we had to re-home our pet cat. What might be a good replacement?

A   *Sadly there are no 'non-allergenic' breeds of dogs or cats. Having small furry pets such as rabbits, guinea pigs or hamsters may work for a short while, but in time allergies to these may develop too, as small animals produce allergen in their urine, which can escape into the air. A chinchilla may be a good option since there are very few reports of confirmed chinchilla allergy. Failing this, try keeping fish.*

9

Chemical attack

Throughout the day, potentially harmful substances threaten us. They have the power to inflame any situation, so here's how to create your own peacekeeping force.

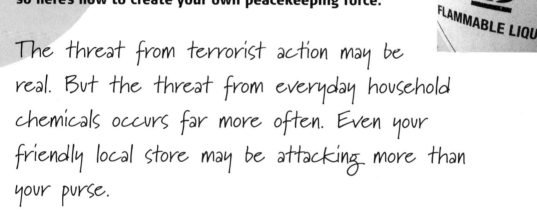

The threat from terrorist action may be real. But the threat from everyday household chemicals occurs far more often. Even your friendly local store may be attacking more than your purse.

Many people are sensitive to chemicals and if they come into contact with them swollen red eyes, nasal congestion or itchy skin may be the outcome. More serious reactions involve asthma symptoms being triggered or a full-blown anaphylactic reaction developing. So if chemicals may cause you problems, you need to avoid them – and this is where you need a bag full of avoidance tactics.

Walking through a department store should be one of the most relaxing experiences on the high street. Soothing music wafts from hidden speakers, and numerous products offer the chance of some serious retail therapy. OK, so before

Here's an idea for you...

Write down what may irritate you if you come into contact with it, for example, nickel, detergents or other chemicals. Now create a strategy to avoid them. For example, if you react to the chemical used to clean computer keyboards, leave a clearly visible note on your keyboard asking for it not to be cleaned. If you are sensitive to detergents in regular soaps, carry your own soap with you. This way you'll be less likely to become irritated and will get more pleasure from what you are doing.

Christmas and in the New Year sales these stores may be packed, but even then the adrenaline rush and the buzz of getting the bargain makes it all worthwhile. It does until you are attacked, that is. Yes, you read that right: attacked. Not by other shoppers reaching for the same bargain as you, but by store employees trying to sell you their wares.

I use the word 'attacked' because that's what it feels like when, just inside the store, the young lady or gentleman moves towards you and before they have finished asking 'Would you like to try our new "Eau de Bull" spray, sir?' their twitching index finger has depressed the button and you're engulfed in a fine mist of their product. But it's not only perfume that can irritate people, although it's one of the commonest irritants, especially if you buy your new girlfriend or boyfriend the wrong one. Cigarette smoke, petrol fumes, smog, pollen or substances that you use in your work can be irritating too, and so avoid them you must.

To achieve this you need a strategy. For example, if you're allergic to pollen, wearing shades and a mask that covers your nose and mouth will help prevent pollen getting into your system. Using the store attack scenario as an example of how to avoid chemical irritants, the most drastic avoidance measure is that you never attend that store again. But if you like the store, why should you suffer by missing out? Anyway, avoiding the store would mean you had lost the battle, had turned your back and run away. You could go to a different store, but the same thing is likely to happen again.

Having a strategy can help to keep you out of deep water. Try IDEA 10, _Nice big breaths_, to find out how a few deep breaths can do the same.

Try another idea...

What do armed forces do when they want get in somewhere without being noticed? They use a 'back door', which is exactly what you could do, provided it isn't also patrolled by freelance beauty product sellers. Of course, you could always use a few choice phrases to see the offending salesperson off, but this would probably get you forcibly removed from the store and set off your allergy symptoms into the bargain. But some less earthy verbal deterrents, such as 'I'm allergic' or 'I'm sensitive', usually do the job – especially now the world is so litigious.

These unprovoked store attacks used to irritate me, not physically, unless the perpetrators decided that the only way to persuade me to buy was to spray the offending substance into my eyes, but it would wind me up. And I had every right to be wound up. It spoiled my relaxing experience, and made my heart start pounding before I'd even got anywhere near the ladies' lingerie department. But I don't get wound up any more. Instead, I treat avoiding these irritating triggers as a game, like tag or touch rugby, and I enjoy playing to win.

'**Not all chemicals are bad. Without hydrogen or oxygen, for example, there would be no way to make water, a vital ingredient in beer.'**
DAVE BARRY

Defining idea...

How did
it go?

**Q   I know it's a good idea to wear shades and a mask, but I can
hardly do this in winter, can I?**

A   *If you don't feel comfortable wearing these, why not try wearing a scarf
around your mouth and nose? Although not as good as a mask, it will offer
some protection, and will also keep you warm! If you don't wear prescription
glasses, a pair of non-prescription glasses with clear lenses will also provide
some protection.*

**Q   I'm a non-smoker and my workplace is no smoking, but when my
smoking colleagues return after having a cigarette the smell of the
smoke gets to me. Any tips?**

A   *Aromatherapy oils effectively overcome the smell of smoke. Why do you
think your parents' house was always filled with lavender after a dinner
party? To disguise the smell left by cigars! Make sure that you or your
colleagues are not sensitive to the fragrances first, though, otherwise you
could have a whole new problem on your hands.*

**Q   I'm failing miserably in the department store department. I always
get sprayed. What can I do, as I enjoy shopping there?**

A   *When I was a child I used to play a game called 'British Bulldogs', which
entailed running from one end of the playground to the other whilst
avoiding those trying to catch you. Well, try this when you enter the store.
Watch the assistant's movements and sell her dummies or sidestep her. Do
whatever it takes, within reason. Another idea is to become the shadow of
another customer so that they get caught by the assistant and you don't.
You see, it can actually be quite good fun after all.*

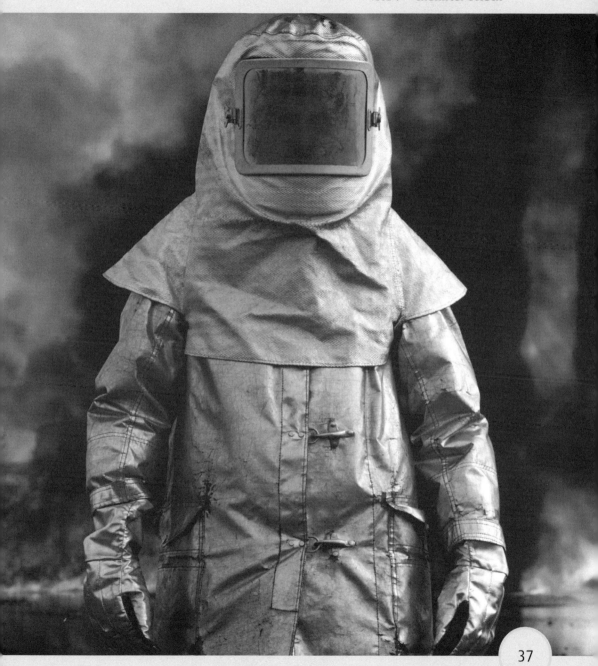

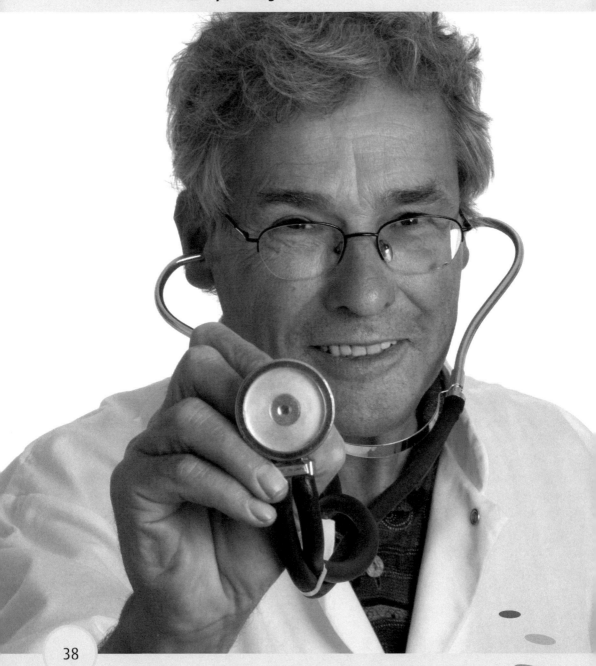

10

Nice big breaths

A slip of the tongue can get you into deep water, but these deep breaths can get you out of trouble.

Picture the scene. A male doctor is in the process of listening to the chest of a buxom woman. 'Nice big breaths', he instructs. 'Thank-you', she replies.

It's one of the oldest sketches in medical humour, but they say the old ones are the best. Nowadays, however, this kind of misunderstanding is more likely to leave the doctor nursing a slapped cheek and not the traditional grin of approval for his cheekiness. But relaxing deep breathing exercises are simple and effective for calming the mind and body, and help keep allergy symptoms under control too.

When we feel stressed or anxious, perhaps because our itchy skin won't give us a moment's peace or, through asthma or hayfever, there's tightness in our chest that's making us feel like we can't breathe, our breathing automatically becomes rapid and shallow. This creates a negative downward spiral. Stress and anxiety increase, in turn causing the symptoms being experienced to intensify, which further increases stress and anxiety, and so on.

39

Here's an idea for you... **Lie on your back with the palms of your hands turned upwards and your feet turned outwards. Concentrate on breathing in through your nose and then out through your mouth. Slowly breathe in and out, concentrating on each breath, and do this for about 15 minutes. You'll quickly discover how easy it is to do, and how much more relaxed and controlled you and your breathing are.**

So what needs to happen? First you need to calm down. Don't shout at me. I know you know this, but shouting is only going to increase your stress and anxiety, which isn't what we want. We want those anxiety and stress levels to fall because this will enable your mind and body to focus clearly and effectively. I'm trying to help you reduce your nervousness here. Why? Well, because I like you, and because when we are nervous, we have trouble learning, remembering and integrating new strategies into our lives – and I want you to get hold of this idea and use it!

You see, when you relax a little your overall feelings of stress, anxiety and even panic will subside. Being told to 'pull yourself together' is just not going to cut it – you already know you should try and do this, and don't need some smart-arse telling you. But even if you wanted to, you couldn't do it anyway. Why? Because during these moments of uncontrolled stress our ability to rationalise and think clearly becomes diminished. Consequently this exacerbates the problem.

However, 'take a few deep breaths' is something that anyone in this situation should be happy to hear, and to have help with, because it works. Deep breathing exercises that relax the mind and body are the foundation of many different therapies and practices, such as stress management, yoga and Tai Chi. They help focus the mind and get more oxygen into the blood stream. For example the

Russian scientist Konstantin Buteyko has developed and promoted the Buteyko technique of breathing to help those with asthma. His theory is that asthma is caused by hyperventilation and this has led him to devise a system of breathing exercises designed to return breathing to normal levels. Other experts in the field of asthma have suggested that Buteyko breathing exercises can improve asthma symptoms in some people, and there is some research to support this belief. However, it is important to recognise that it does not provide a cure for asthma but, used alongside conventional asthma treatment, it may help some people to cope better with their symptoms.

Breathing exercises are easy to do and can be done pretty much anywhere you fancy or find yourself. They help regulate the breathing and calm a stressed mind. It's important to try and concentrate on breathing from the abdomen as the ribcage expands, since this helps to ensure that the deepest breaths are taken. It's a bit easier to do if you put a hand on your abdomen so you can feel your stomach area rise as your diaphragm and ribcage expand. Oh, and remember to put yourself in a warm, safe and comfortable position too.

Try another idea...

Now you've got the hang of relaxing breathing, breeze away to IDEA 26, Rubber rising, to get a grip on preventing unwanted swellings from taking over.

Defining idea...

'As we free our breath (through diaphragmatic breathing) we relax our emotions and let go our body tensions.'
GAY HENDRICKS, psychologist and author

41

How did
it go?

Q **Do I have to do it lying down or can I do it in any other position?**

A   *Most people start off practising deep breathing relaxation exercises by lying down, since lying down is relaxing in itself. But you can also practise these exercises whilst standing or sitting. Whether you stand or sit, ensure that you are upright and not slouched, so you have the best chance of getting plenty of air into the lungs.*

Q **I've heard about nasal breathing exercises. Are these any good?**

A   *They can help, and can be done as follows. Close the right nostril with your thumb and breathe out through your left nostril. Next breathe in through your left nostril for a count of four, and then close both nostrils and hold the breath for a count of ten. Now, keeping your left nostril closed, breathe out through your right nostril and then in through it for a count of four again. Close both nostrils and count to ten then, keeping the right nostril closed, breathe out from the left again.*

Q **How often should I do deep breathing exercises?**

A   *Doing them every few hours throughout the day will help you to keep unwanted stress under control and give you plenty of opportunity to practise so that you build up your confidence in your ability to relax yourself whenever you need to. If you continue practising breathing this way you'll soon be doing it naturally throughout the day. Alternatively you can just do them when you find yourself stressed and anxious to help overcome the stress you're experiencing.*

11

A dose of sea air

Donkey rides, buckets and spades, the smell of the ocean. We all feel better at the seaside. But you don't have to be anywhere near the sea to get the benefits. Here's how to reap the rewards no matter where you live.

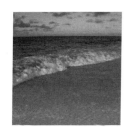

Banish thoughts of rain and wind, overcoats, and people huddled in the shelter overlooking a deserted beach. Just think about the good things the seaside brings.

Ice creams, deckchairs, seafood and all the fun of the fair. It's safe for you to leave your handkerchief knotted on your head too, because with a little dose of sea air your nose will be as clear as a mariner's bell.

Just thinking about a trip to the seaside helps your mind to relax. You feel happy because it probably brings back many wonderful childhood memories – unless your overwhelming memory is of being lost and waiting in the beach inspector's office whilst he tried to summon your parents over the public address system. If you are relaxed you are less likely to suffer the symptoms of your specific allergy; and if you do, at least you'll be in a better frame of mind to deal with them. But there's more to the seaside than this.

Here's an idea for you... **Make a trip to the seaside. Walk along the beach or the seafront taking nice deep breaths in and out and feel how much easier your breathing becomes. Alternatively go along to your local pharmacy and buy a seawater micro-diffusion nasal spray and enjoy the benefits of the seaside in the comfort of your own home.**

For centuries the benefits of sea water have been recognised, with people flocking to the sea to 'take of the water'. Remember those photographs of men and women leaving the bathing huts with their trousers and skirts hitched up to go paddling? Perhaps they had a point, keeping all those clothes on: nowadays, it's more a case of strip off, rush into the sea – and rush back out again as soon as the cold water reaches the more sensitive parts!

Why a dose of sea air is good for the nostrils is down to the microscopic drops of liquid and their contents. The moisture that 'gets up your nose' as you breathe in helps to clear the nose of debris, such as pollen, and the excess mucus that has been produced in response to the allergic stimulus. If you've ever tried learning to water-ski and taken a dive face first, you'll know precisely how well the sea water can flush out the nasal passages! Also, because it's cooler at the coast there's less pollen around to cause problems. Plus in coastal areas pollen is more easily dispersed as sea breezes blow it inland.

Cleaning the nose and lessening the congestion in it allows the nose to function more effectively in filtering out pollen and other allergy symptom triggering irritants that are present in the air breathed in. Moreover, trace elements in the sea water are believed to have specific roles too. For example, manganese, copper and magnesium are thought to be able to relieve and prevent the symptoms of nasal allergy – congestion, running and swelling – through their anti-allergy and anti-inflammatory actions. And further, once your nose is clean, any allergy nasal sprays used will be able to work more effectively too.

So that's got that all cleared up then. Along you go to IDEA 3, *Intolerable cruelty*, and let's clear up a common misconception.

Try another idea...

No, you don't need to move to the coast to reap the benefits, not unless this is just the excuse you've been looking for. You can get at least some of the same benefits wherever you live. To begin with, you can always think about the seaside and remind yourself about how nice it is with photographs or TV programmes. Plus you can have sea water up your nose wherever you are, because sea water micro-sprays are now available that – yes, you've guessed it – contains real sea water and can be sprayed gently into each nostril. This is courtesy of the French, who for a long time have enjoyed the benefits of nasal hygiene, whether it's to help with hayfever, nasal congestion or snoring. As you can see, it's not just ships that come in a bottle – now sea water does, too.

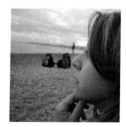 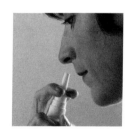

'The cure for anything is salt water: sweat, tears or the sea.'
ISAK DINESEN, Danish author

Defining idea...

45

How did it go?

Q **I have perennial rhinitis, so I suffer with a blocked up nose for most of the year. Could sea water help me?**

A *Yes, using sea water can help in the same way that it helps those with hayfever – by relieving the congestion and removing any irritants from the nostrils.*

Q **How is the sea water nasal spray made and where can I get it?**

A *Sea water is collected from the sea and checked for purity before being taken to the manufacturing plant, where it is checked again, diluted, put into a can and sealed. It's available from pharmacists without a prescription.*

Q **I don't like putting things up my nose. What can I do?**

A *You can always spray the sea water from just outside the nostrils, since often it's the nozzle that bothers people rather than the contents of the spray. An alternative for you may be to boil some water, place it in a bowl and inhale the steam. This will relieve congestion, especially if you add a few drops of eucalyptus, menthol or olbas oil to it. Placing a towel over your head will help keep the steam closer for longer, so will give the greatest benefit.*

Q **How can I make my own?**

A *Make up your own saline (salt water) nose drops mixture by adding half a teaspoon of salt to 250 ml water – don't make it stronger than this as very salty water is unpleasant when put into the nose. Use a dropper to gently drip a couple of drops into each nostril so that the mucus is thinned and, together with any irritants, easily cleared from the nose.*

12

Keep it local

A spoonful of sugar may help the medicine go down, but a spoonful of honey helps soothe all sorts of ailments too. Find out how supporting your community bees may help your allergies at the same time.

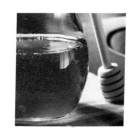

Bees are clever little things. If a bee finds a particularly good source of nectar, it flies the shortest route back to the hive — hence the term 'beeline'.

Bees are also very generous and tell the other bees where to find the nectar by performing a dance routine. If you suffer with hayfever you could gain from being generous and clever too, by buying and enjoying some of their delicious produce.

If it hurts when you bang your head against the wall, you don't keep on doing it, do you? No, you stop it, since this way the pain should go away. Or you avoid doing it in the first place. This is the most basic principle of keeping free of allergy symptoms too if you're susceptible. For example, if it's a particular food that sets you off, then it's best to keep it at arm's length, or in the packet. Likewise, if granny's cats play havoc with your breathing, then keeping away from them is a good idea.

Here's an idea for you...

Get yourself a jar of honey that has been made local to where you live. Have a teaspoonful each day, either neat, mixed with warm water or added to your breakfast cereal. Doing this, you'll be getting a tasty treat and your hayfever may become a thing of the past.

Hayfever is the same. Well almost. Pollen sets your eyes and nose running, so you are advised to avoid it. That's the mantra. Stay out of its way the best you can. Protect yourself by whatever means – shades, sprays, staying indoors if necessary. But what would you say if I told you to eat it? You'd probably think I was mad and want to have me committed. Fair enough – pollen causes your symptoms and I want you to have some. If I'm not mad, then I must be cruel.

So how does honey help with hayfever? It's still not precisely understood, but popular belief goes something like this. The pollen that jumps up your nose and into your eyes when you go outdoors – that is, the pollen local to where you live – is often the main trigger for your hayfever attack. Locally made honey likewise contains these irritating pollens, caught up in the nectar collected by the bees. It's believed that giving the body a regular tiny dose of these pollens, the ones that upset you, helps the body build resistance to their effects by teaching it not to react to them. So, when the hayfever season arrives and pollen is all around, the body is already prepared and protected. It's a similar principle to the process of desensitising people by giving them injections of the specific pollen they are allergic to – only using a spoon, not a needle. So a daily teaspoon of locally produced honey could help keep your hayfever symptoms at bay.

Awareness of the benefits of honey is not new. Honey was one of the most common ingredients in medicines in Ancient Egypt and has been used for centuries to benefit health.

Slip along to **IDEA 51, *Dad's Daily Dose*, and have a taste of dad's favourite recipe.**

Try another idea...

Honey can help to fight infection because of its antibacterial properties, and it's often used to treat burns and open wounds. More recently researchers from New Zealand have suggested that honey made from the manuka flower could be used to treat stomach ulcers. Honey is a good cure for hangovers, too, since its high content of sugar helps to speed up the processing of alcohol by the liver. It's also a good general pick-me-up.

So enjoy your honey and consider this. If you think that you cover a lot of miles in your job then spare a thought for the bees, who will have to fly about 55,000 miles to make just one pound of honey.

'The only reason for being a bee is to make honey. And the only reason for making honey is so I can eat it.'
WINNIE THE POOH

Defining idea...

Q   Does the honey have to be locally made?

How did it go?

A   *Yes, it does. It's believed that to be effective in controlling hayfever symptoms the honey must be produced locally, and ideally within a ten mile radius of your home. However, even if the honey is produced outside this area it's still worth giving it a try.*

49

Q   **I can't find any locally made honey in my local foodstore. Is there anywhere else I could try?**

A   *Local farmer's markets and country shows are good places to start. Ask around or put an advert in the newsagent's window. In most areas there are usually people who keep bees as a hobby who'll be happy to tell you about bee keeping and sell you some of their honey. They may even encourage you to take up the hobby – which, if you can't find any locally produced honey, may be the best alternative. Your national or regional beekeepers association should keep a list of beekeepers in your area. In the UK, for example, visit the British Beekeepers Association's website at http://www.bbka.org.uk*

Q   **How come if you eat the pollen it doesn't cause hayfever symptoms?**

A   *When you breathe in pollen that you are sensitive to your body reacts by attacking it and defending itself since it sees the pollen as a foreign invader looking to cause trouble. However, when these substances are consumed the body doesn't usually mount this sort of attack against them and in time, as consequence of this, it may become acclimatised to the pollen.*

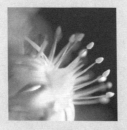

13

Ah, what a relief

If your eyes are running, your skin is itching or you can't stop sneezing, then reach for something to ease the misery. There's a host of things to choose from, so take a dip into your armoury.

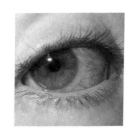

Maybe you'd rather not suffer at all?
What do I mean, maybe? Of course you'd rather not be put through all this.

Allergies could be likened to football hooliganism. You see the substances that trigger an allergy attack are actually harmless, like the innocent football supporters of the visiting team who just want to watch their team play. For those who are allergic, it's their body's inappropriate overreaction to these visitors that's the problem, like the football hooligans who are intent on having a go. What's happening is that certain substances, for example pollen or house dust mite dung, are seen by the body as being dangerous. Why? Because the body has been inappropriately conditioned to respond in this way. When it encounters them, rather than just getting on with what it's doing and letting them get on with what they're doing, it gets angry, flares up, and causes trouble and misery.

Here's an idea for you...

The most important part of controlling allergies is avoiding the allergy trigger as best you can, but medicines are important too. The reality is that many people only make a half-hearted attempt to use their medicines and often use them incorrectly, so get little or no benefit. Try following your allergy medicine instructions to the letter. Doing this gives you the best chance of feeling better.

So what's the solution? Well, it's not possible to cure allergies – not yet, anyway. But they can be kept under control such that they don't play up, or at least so that when they do you can quickly gain the upper hand.

Let's imagine that you're a hayfever sufferer and that pollen and your body are two football teams from the same city. It's derby day. Now it may not be possible to prevent the supporters of these two teams from being exposed to each other, but it is possible to take steps to minimise the risks and the amount of harm that occurs.

To begin with, you need to keep the two factions away from each other. But this is easier said than done. During the hayfever season, for example, pollen is always around, and even though on a particular day the forecast may say the count is low, you may still be exposed to it. Likewise on match-day there's always the chance that the odd fan will slip through the net and into the lion's den and stir up trouble. Fortunately there are many ways to relieve or prevent trouble.

One way is to put a ring around the group of fans to prevent them from reaching the opposition's area, for example. Mast-cell-stabilising drugs, or cromoglycate-like drugs, act like this by stabilising the outer membrane of the mast cell (the cell containing allergy-triggering chemicals like histamine) and hence preventing its contents from escaping.

Another option is to put a police block in the way so one can't get to the other. This is how antihistamines work. Marvellous drugs that, although rarely used to treat asthma or eczema because they have very little beneficial effect on these allergies, are great for treating hayfever, perennial allergic rhinitis and chronic urticaria. Histamine is the chemical responsible for much of the misery of allergies, and it does so by attaching itself to specific receptors in the body. Antihistamines, which come as nasal sprays, eye drops, tablets and creams, also attach to these receptors, and if they get there first they'll prevent histamine from doing so.

Spraying water on something, or somebody, is a very good way of diffusing and calming down a volatile situation – except in wet T-shirt competitions, where it's designed to have the opposite effect! Sometimes it can prevent problems progressing when trouble has already started, like when opposing fans have already made contact with each other. Some drugs, for example steroids contained in nasal sprays, creams and inhalers, play a similar role to this. Like the high-pressure water jet, their effect can be targeted to where it's needed. If this is the lungs, then an inhaler is used; if it's the nose, then nasal sprays or drops are used. The advantage of this is that other parts of the body, the innocent bystanders in T-shirts for example, are less likely to suffer the side effects.

Try another idea…

Steroids are often used to help keep allergies under control. Take a big breath and try IDEA 14, *Steroid phobia*, to uncover the truth about these drugs.

Defining idea…

'Though no one can go back and make a brand new start, anyone can start from now and make a brand new ending.'
CARL BARD

53

How did it go?

Q When's the best time to take antihistamines?

A   It's best to take them well before trouble is likely to begin. Antihistamines can't knock histamine off the receptor once it has attached itself, so to work they need to get onto the receptor before the histamine does. Taking antihistamines at the first sign of symptoms will still be of some benefit, but not to the same extent as taking it beforehand. With hayfever it's best to start taking them a couple of weeks before the pollen season starts, and then continue taking them throughout the season.

Q How do antileukotriene drugs work?

A   Leukotrienes are some of the chemicals that are produced by mast cells during an allergic reaction. They are messenger chemicals and attract more immune cells to the part of the body where the allergic reaction is taking place. In school playgrounds the kid who shouts 'scrap!' when a fight starts would be their equivalent; in a political demonstration they'd be the one who phones for additional supporters to come and join in the fight. Some antileukotriene drugs work by preventing leukotrienes from attaching to their target and so prevent perpetuation of the inflammation process, whilst others work by blocking leukotriene production altogether.

Q What about decongestants?

A   Decongestants are an effective way to relieve a stuffy nose, a common symptom of hayfever and of allergies to dust and pets. Available as tablets, capsules, nasal sprays or liquids, they can be used to disperse irritations effectively.

14

Steroid phobia

Headlines are always appearing about how steroids did this, steroids did that – and in the tabloids, how steroids did the other too. Let's see how they can calm down even the most inflamed situations.

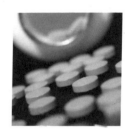

Very few drugs have had such a bad press as steroids. As far as the medical profession is concerned, the fear this publicity has created amongst the public is now commonly known as 'steroid phobia'.

Let's get one thing clear from the start. When medical doctors talk about steroids we are not talking about those drugs that people abuse to enhance their athletic performance, that contribute to frighteningly large collar sizes and make ordinary looking female athletes look like, well, you know what I mean. We're talking about the drugs that are similar to cortisol, a steroid that the body makes naturally and that is essential if the body is to fight stress, injury and disease effectively. Yes, you read that correctly, the body makes its own steroid. Or, to administer it in tabloid form, 'Shock horror! Body makes steroid!'

If you've been put off steroids by lurid newspaper stories, think back to how you felt when you were using them. Depending on your allergy, there's a very good chance that you were breathing more easily, you had fewer asthma attacks, your nose felt clear, you didn't sneeze so much, or your skin looked healthy and didn't itch. Provided your doctor confirms it's OK to do so, give them another chance and feel the difference.

The most important action of the corticosteroid drugs used in medicine is to reduce the inflammation that's associated with medical conditions such as allergies, inflammatory bowel disease and arthritis. They are also used to suppress the body's immune response, for example, to reduce the chance of rejection in patients who have received organ transplants. Now if this still doesn't provide a positive headline about steroids, perhaps hinting that they can enhance your sex life will. I know what you're thinking: how can something that *reduces* swelling improve sex? Surely that can't be right?

Let's take asthma as an example. Inflammation of the inner lining of the airways in the lungs is the major cause of asthma symptoms – chest tightness, wheezing and shortness of breath. Have you ever tried to kiss when you can't breathe easily? Well, it's not easy. It's barely possible to make love if you can't breathe clearly either. The use of steroids, which are usually administered via an inhaler, helps to keep the lungs less inflamed and consequently keep those with asthma free of symptoms. Ah, it's beginning to make sense isn't it? In eczema the skin becomes dry and itchy. You scratch it and this causes the release of chemicals that trigger inflammation and more itch, and so the cycle continues. You may not want anyone else to see your skin, let alone touch it for fear of making it worse, so sex may be less likely when you've got a flare-up. And if your eyes are watering and your nose is blocked because of hayfever, you're hardly going to feel in the mood, now are you?

So here's a possible headline – 'Allergy sufferer uses steroids for sex romp'. Or, more realistically, by keeping allergy symptoms under control, steroids may well improve your sex life.

Now you've stripped away the myths about steroids it's time for you to try IDEA 15, *Let's get naked*.

Try another idea...

I'm not saying that steroids don't have any risk of side effects: they do. There's a risk of side effects with all drugs. And, as with all drugs, the side effects of steroids are most common when they are taken for prolonged periods and in very high doses. For this reason, when doctors prescribe steroids they do so in the lowest dose and for the shortest period of time. Some people, for example those with asthma, need to use a steroid inhaler on a daily basis to keep their symptoms under control. Those with hayfever may find they need to use their steroid nasal spray throughout the hayfever season. The fact that usually the dose administered is the lowest that will successfully do the job and the fact that it is being targeted at the relevant part of the body ensure that the risk of side effects is kept to a minimum. And it's important not to forget why steroids are prescribed in the first place. And no, it's not about sex – well, not only sex. It's about good old-fashioned quality of life. Whether they be in creams, inhalers or nasal sprays, steroids can give people their quality of life back. Now, that really is a headline.

'Only the suppressed word is dangerous.'
LUDWIG BORNE, German journalist

Defining idea...

How did it go?

Q **Is there an alternative to using steroids for my rhinitis? I really don't want to use them?**

A *The advantage of steroid nose drops and sprays is that they can be used as a preventative to stop inflammation in the first place or as a treatment to stop it developing any further. However, there are a number of alternatives. Cromoglycate-like drugs will prevent the allergic reaction before it starts, and antihistamines block the process before inflammation gets going.*

Q **Will taking steroids for my asthma make me look like a weightlifter?**

A *No. The steroids used to help treat people with allergies, and those with other inflammatory conditions for that matter, are called corticosteroids and are similar to the natural steroid hormone produced by the body. It's anabolic steroids that are misused to pump up muscles artificially. Although the term 'steroids' is often used when talking about both types, they really are very different.*

Q **My doctor prescribes me a combination of steroid and antibiotic cream to treat my eczema when it flares up. Why is this?**

A *Not long ago research found that very often the trigger for eczema flare-up is a bacterium called Staphylococcus aureus that normally lives on the skin. For those with eczema, if the bacterium gets into the skin through cracks or when scratching it can trigger a flare-up. Treatment with an antibiotic not only eliminates the bacteria and helps the skin to recover, but since the bacteria hamper the effectiveness of steroids, eliminating them also helps the steroid cream to work better. This means that lower strengths of steroid are needed to bring the eczema under control.*

15

Let's get naked

Indoor naturism may entertain your neighbours if you live in a glasshouse or forget to draw the curtains, but it can bring enormous amounts of pleasure for hayfever sufferers too. Here's how.

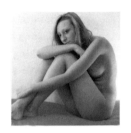

Once you're through your front door after a hard day's work, off come your coat and shoes, and up the stairs you go. In your bedroom you change into something more comfortable.

Sound familiar? It's what many people do, but if you're an allergy sufferer, particularly a hayfever sufferer, this kind of behaviour is going to cause you problems. You see, pollen is sticky and likes to stick around. Even though it may not be easy to see them you can guarantee that millions of tiny grains of pollen, like in the Lionel Richie song, are stuck on you. So this is how you lose these irritating hangers on.

Here's an idea for you... **Keep a rubbish bin liner by the front door to put your clothes in once you strip off. Take your clothes in the bin liner to the washing machine. Once you've emptied the liner, throw it away. By doing this you'll reduce the chances of pollen getting around your home.**

Even if you don't have hayfever yourself, you're bound to know someone who has it. Sometimes first thing in the morning the person with hayfever will look awful. And not because they've had a night on the tiles – well, not necessarily – although that is how they'll feel. It's because despite the fact that the night-time is supposed to be a safe haven for hayfever sufferers – unless you're camping out and lying with your head in the grass – they've still had a bad night and feel dreadful.

The reason for this is that if you leave the clothes you've been wearing outdoors in your bedroom, or, worse still, on your bed, you're loading the bedroom up with pollen that overnight is quite literally going to get up your nose. And we all know what happens then. Blocked nose, open mouth, difficulty in breathing...what can be only described as a very unpleasant, and rough, night.

Think about when you come home in the rain. What do you do with your umbrella? You shake it off outside before coming in, maybe even leaving it in the porch to dry off. You certainly wouldn't carry it upstairs to your bedroom, or you might have an embarrassing wet patch on the bed to explain away. If you've been gardening, doing DIY or even mud slinging with your neighbour, again what do you do? You leave your dirty boots and clothes somewhere where the dirt isn't going to get trampled through the house. Remember your mother shouting at you for doing that! You leave the clothes in the laundry room, for instance, or bung them straight into the washing machine.

Well, it should be no different with pollen and hayfever. In fact, you should take it one step further. The moment you get through the door, strip off. Don't wait until you get upstairs into your bedroom or your bathroom, just get your kit off as soon as you enter the house. Make sure you close the door first, though. After all, you wouldn't want to cause a bad reaction with any of the neighbours who might spot you – that would be rash. By stripping off you've left the pollen away from the parts of your home where you are going to spend the rest of the day. All this could still be to no avail, however, because, like sand, pollen gets everywhere. It'll be stuck in your hair and on your hands too, so will need to be washed off. Go and have a shower, preferably a cold one, because with all the excitement of getting naked in a new and semi-public place you're going to need to cool off.

So there you have it. You have a genuinely valid reason for behaving as though you're in the movie *9 1/2 weeks*. Well, perhaps the first fortnight, anyway.

Try another idea...

Now you know how to avoid spreading pollen around your home, have a gander at IDEA 16, *Dust to dust*, to see how to keep your home clear of other allergens too.

Defining idea...

'When you find a burden in belief or apparel, cast it off.'
AMELIA BLOOMER, 1850s proponent of women's equality and body acceptance.

61

Q **I have a glass front door. What can I do?**

A *Try undressing just to the side of the door. Perhaps it's easier for you to come in through the back door instead. Just make sure that you strip off in the same place every time, ideally somewhere where you wouldn't usually stand or sit. This way, any pollen that comes off your clothing is likely to remain in this place and not get transferred around your home.*

Q **Can't I just throw my clothes into my usual dirty laundry basket?**

A *Yes, you can do this if you prefer, since the next stop for clothing from here is the washing machine – unless you're a student, that is! The problem is that some pollen will attach itself to the basket itself and therefore may find its way back onto you. Many people have their dirty laundry basket in close proximity to clean clothing so once again pollen transfer may occur from clothes worn outdoor clothes to other clothes.*

Q **I've tried stripping off but I'm still getting symptoms of hayfever at night. Am I missing something?**

A *Pollen must be getting to you via some other means. In your hair, on your hands, or perhaps on your dog if you have one. Other people in your household may be bringing it in on their clothing, so try to get them to strip and shower when they come home. That should be easy, provided you don't all arrive at the same time!*

16

Dust to dust

Here's why giving your home a good going over with the vacuum cleaner not only puts the freshness back, it evicts unwanted guests that trigger allergy symptoms too.

Some people love to vacuum, others simply loathe it. There's no escape because, one way or another, if you're to avoid being up to your neck in dust and allergy symptoms it has to be done.

Many people find vacuuming relaxing. I'm not joking. The gentle movement and humming can be very soothing, for babies in particular. Of course, vacuuming is a very important way of keeping allergy-triggering substances, or allergens, to a minimum, so that there is less chance of them causing you problems.

Personally, I don't mind vacuuming. I'd rather do it than the ironing, for instance. I find it relaxing since whilst I'm making my way around the house I listen to music. It's an opportunity to do some exercise and to do something that I really enjoy (that's the listening to music, which is something I don't have the time to do as much I'd like). OK, so I don't vacuum as often as I used to because I now have a

Here's an idea for you...

When you vacuum, cover any furniture, especially the bed and soft furniture, with a clean sheet and leave at least one window open in each room being vacuumed. Once you have finished, leave the windows open for 30 minutes, and after closing the windows leave the sheets in place for another 30 minutes. Then carefully remove the sheets from the furniture. This will reduce the amount of dust that resettles on the furniture and that you will be exposed to.

cleaner – for allergy sufferers the best solution is to let someone else do the vacuuming – but when I do have to vacuum it's easier to see it as an opportunity than a chore.

It's not only the floors and carpets that need doing. House dust mites and their dung also congregate in mattresses and furniture, so these will need to be vacuumed too. And this needs to be done at least once a week if you suffer with indoor allergies.

Vacuuming can be good for your overall health too. In order keep your weight at a healthy level and keep your heart fit, at least 30 minutes of moderately intensive activity on at least five days a week is recommended. Alternatively, you could try to take 10,000 steps a day. Housework, such as washing the windows, can be used as part of this daily exercise quota. Vacuuming in particular can count as a moderately intensive exercise when you put some effort into it. And it's cheaper than going to the gym.

One of the problems with vacuum cleaning is that a fair amount of the dust, house dust mites and other allergens that get sucked into the vacuum machine are then sprayed out again through the vacuum cleaner's exhaust. This is why dusting is best done with a damp cloth – the dust collects on the cloth rather than just being wafted into the air.

With regards to allergy control, there's little point vacuuming if all you are doing is sending the allergen elsewhere in the room. It's here that modern technology has come to the rescue.

So vacuuming can be less painful than you thought. Try IDEA 44, *'ello Vera*, to see how this wonderful plant can ease your troubles.

Try another idea...

Contamination control has always been important in many walks of life. For example, many years ago Swiss watchmakers covered their sensitive timepieces with a small bell jar to prevent dust from falling on them when they were not being worked on. For allergy control it's vitally important that house dust mites and other allergenic particles, once sucked up into the vacuum cleaner, are prevented from leaving it again. Probably the most effective way of controlling this is the HEPA (High Efficiency Particulate Air) filter, which is now incorporated into many different vacuum cleaners and room air purifiers. HEPA filters retain 99.9% of particles in the range of 0.3 to 0.5 microns and will retain house dust mites, mould and animal allergens. Vacuum cleaners with HEPA filters have helped to make life much more comfortable for many allergy sufferers.

Whether you use a streamlined vacuum cleaner that looks like a work of art or one that looks like a throwback to an old sci-fi B movie, it doesn't matter. Just be sure to put some effort into it, keep on sucking and don't forget the corners.

'When your dreams turn to dust, vacuum.'
ANONYMOUS

Defining idea...

How did it go?

Q   Some of my rooms don't have windows. What can I do?

A   *Make sure that you keep the door open to allow some ventilation when you are vacuuming. A good idea if you find vacuuming upsets your allergies, or you simply hate the thought of vacuuming, is to try using a dehumidifier. Some of these are actually designed to kill mites since they reduce the humidity to levels where the mites dry out and die.*

Q   I'd like a vacuum cleaner with a HEPA filter but they're very expensive. Any tips for me?

A   *First of all, when you dust make sure you use a damp cloth. Try adding some eucalyptus oil to the cloth as this can deter mites. Anti-mite dusters are available that have an electrostatic charge to hold the dust, so think about trying one of these. When it's time to empty the bag in your vacuum cleaner always do this outside, and if possible ask someone else to do this for you. Whilst vacuuming try wearing a cycle or other mask.*

Q   I know it's important to vacuum regularly, but it's such a chore. How can I get round this?

A   *You could employ someone else to do it, or you could take steps to make it less of a punishment. Imagine being a racing driver when you vacuum, or being on an off-road 4x4 track. Think safety first so you don't injure anyone around you. Another popular activity is air-guitaring with the vacuum hose. If you find it's the air that's getting vacuumed but not the carpets, try dancing whilst you vacuum instead.*

17

Water, water everywhere

It's good to keep the body hydrated throughout the day. But drinking it isn't the only way to help ease the symptoms of allergy.

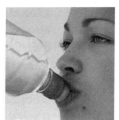

Water makes up about 70% of an adult's body weight and covers nearly 140 million square miles of the earth's surface. No life can exist without it, and that includes you.

It's a good thing there's so much of it about, since without it we would die within a matter of days. Water helps the body digest food and remove waste products, it keeps our joints and eyes well lubricated, and it helps regulate body temperature. But on an average day we lose around two litres of water when we breathe, in waste products and through sweat, and this needs to be replaced. Replacing it helps to control allergy symptoms too. For example, water keeps the skin supple making it less likely to become dry, cracked, and itchy as it does in those with eczema. Making the environment a little misty helps keep the mucous membranes and tiny hair cells that line the nose in good condition, so they can function properly too.

Here's an idea for you...

Try short bursts of increased humidity. You don't have to use a humidifier. Take a bowl of warm water and, making sure that it's safe to do this, just place it near the radiator. If you are in the kitchen, put a saucepan of water on the stove; if you spend hours sitting on the toilet or preening yourself in the bathroom, run the hot taps of the bath or run a hot shower for a while. By increasing the humidity in these ways your skin, eyes and nose should feel much clearer.

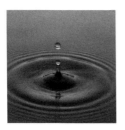

Air-conditioning and central heating can create a very dry environment. Consequently everything becomes dry. Have you noticed how dry your skin is and how dry your mouth feels when you're in this kind of environment? Many people with allergies find that a little humidification can help. Now, of course, too much humidity contributes to house dust mite proliferation, which won't help those allergic to its dung. Finding the right balance is what's important, so it's a case of sniff it and see.

Many of you will have been in a sauna or steam room. And I'm sure there are lots of tales about the mists clearing to reveal more than you bargained for, but forget that for now. Remember how it felt when you took a deep breath in, having naively added cold water to the coals thinking that it would cool things down? Yes, it may have burned a little in your nostrils, but your nose felt clearer, too, didn't it? Even if you haven't been in a sauna, you'll have been in a hot shower surrounded by steam, and I expect your breathing would have felt much better then, too.

Unless you've won the lottery or have a serious prune-skin fetish, you really can't expect to go in and out of a sauna all day, every day. So, to combat the effects of dry modern-day environments, humidifiers have been developed for home use and are increasingly available to relieve the unpleasant discomfort of dry nose, lips, throat and skin. Although there are many different types, they basically all do the same thing – a bit like politicians, I suppose, but unlike politicians, humidifiers tend to be effective and efficient.

Enjoyed getting moist? Good. Try IDEA 23, *Ooh, that's gonna cost you*, and find out a simple and effective way of unblocking your passages.

Try another idea...

Put simply, all they do is put moisture in the air. It's how they go about achieving this that varies. For instance, the simplest, usually known as a vaporiser, just boils water and sends it into the air as steam. Others will simply blow air through a wet pad so that the air collects moisture as it weaves it's merry way into the room. The impeller flings water at a diffuser, which breaks the water into fine droplets that float into the air. For the more gadget mad amongst you, high-tech ultrasonic versions use a metal diaphragm vibrating at an ultrasonic frequency, much like the element in a high-frequency speaker, to create water droplets.

It actually doesn't really matter how you get the humidity back into a room so long as the way you do it does it for you.

'Water is the best of all things.'
PINDAR

Defining idea...

How did it go?

Q   I have young children at home, so I don't like leaving warm water around if it's not necessary. What should I do?

A   *I agree that this can be a problem. You should always make sure that it is safe before trying any of these ideas. Try using cool water in the bowl near the radiator so if your child did try to get hold of it they should only get a soaking and not hurt. If you are still not sure, you don't have to place it near the radiator. Simply placing a bowl of cool water anywhere in the room will allow some humidification to occur if the room is warm and dry.*

Q   What about wet towels?

A   *Well excuse me, but what you get up to in your own home is entirely up to you! OK, I know – you don't mean flicking people with them. Seriously, yes, wet or damp towels are an excellent way to increase the humidity of a room. Hanging them over a chair near a radiator, for example, should be particularly effective because of their large surface area.*

Q   Can oils help?

A   *Yes, they can – which is why many of the humidifiers available for home use are able to vaporise these oils when they are added to the water. Menthol, olbas or eucalyptus are popular ones and make a room smell nice as well as helping to clear the nostrils.*

18

What's your poison?

Everyone thinks they have a food allergy these days, but what's the truth behind this internal explosion? Here are the facts and fads of food allergy.

People are getting fatter by the day and the obesity crisis is almost out of control. So surely we can't all be allergic to food?

No, of course not, although listening to people around you you'd believe that everyone is. Many like to believe that it's an allergy that's responsible for problems in their life – constant tiredness, weight gain, poor sex life, even not being promoted. Some people think it's fashionable to have an allergy, thanks to celebrities and the media. And if you think that having an allergy is fashionable, then having a food allergy moves you smoothly into the VIP lounge and onto the A-list amongst this crowd.

The reality is that, although food allergy is becoming more common, it's nowhere near as common as people think. However, for those with true food allergy the problem is real, very real.

Here's an idea for you...

Make a list of foods that are safe for you to eat. To make this easier, larger supermarkets often have 'free-from' lists available, as do major food manufacturers. Keep it with you, distribute it to friends and family – even pin it up on the noticeboard at work. By doing this you'll make shopping, cooking and eating much less hassle and you'll be reducing your risk of suffering allergic reactions.

At the mildest end of the spectrum tingling or itching in or around the lips and mouth may be all that happens when the food culprit makes contact. For babies with food allergy their gut is the likely victim, causing vomiting and diarrhoea. Now there's a good reason to keep 'the naughty foods away from oo then'. Symptoms of asthma and eczema may also be triggered by certain foods. At the other end of the spectrum severe allergic, or anaphylactic, reaction, with light-headedness, difficulty breathing, a sense of impending doom, shock and loss of consciousness, puts survival in the hands of immediate emergency treatment. So if you were ever thinking of using food allergy as a reason to escape paying the restaurant bill, think again.

The parts of food responsible for causing allergic reactions, the allergens, are usually proteins. Even after cooking or digestion many of these allergens can still cause reactions. The most common offenders are the proteins in cow's milk, eggs, peanuts, wheat, soy, fish, shellfish and tree nuts. These are responsible for up to 90% of all allergic reactions. In children, the following six foods cause the majority of food allergy reactions: milk, eggs, peanuts, wheat, soy, and tree nuts. In adults, four foods cause the majority of allergic reactions: peanuts, tree nuts, fish and shellfish.

OK, let's take a look at the basics. If you have already been diagnosed with a true food allergy you should know this like the back of your hand, and if you don't then shame on you! If you don't have a food allergy, and I'm talking about a true food allergy, then this is important for you too, because someone around you will have a true food allergy and you need to know what to do if things go pear-shaped.

So you've a good idea what needs to be kept away from you. Now try IDEA 46, *Keeping it out of the family*, to see how to reduce the chances of others in your family getting allergies.

Try another idea...

So step one: avoid the food. Doh! Pretty obvious, even to the Homer Simpsons amongst you. True, but it's not so easy as it sounds. Why? Because the protein responsible may be an ingredient. So step two is to ask about ingredients so that you don't get caught out by hidden food allergens. This is especially important when you are eating away from home since getting caught out when you're playing away can leave you red faced. And if you're the host, don't forget to ask your guests if they have any allergies. Step three: read food labels carefully and get familiar with what the terms used mean. For example, egg white is often listed as albumin, and casein is always made from milk. Hopefully before too long that well-known food manufacturer cop-out, 'may contain traces of ....' will be replaced by something more helpful so that those with food allergy have a greater choice of foods. And so to step four: be prepared for action if an allergic reaction erupts.

'Give me neither poverty nor riches; feed me with food convenient for me.'
PROVERBS 30:8

Defining idea...

How did
it go?

**Q   What should I do when my friend, Al Lergic, comes to stay? I don't
know what foods to avoid.**

*A   Ask him to send you a list of his safe and unsafe foods. Whatever you do,
don't guess. Also ask him to show you what to do if he has a reaction. You,
or anyone around him, be they family, friends or work colleagues, should
know how to use the adrenaline injection, for example. Have a dry run; then
you won't get in a panic if you need to do the real thing. If you are
travelling with your friend, then make sure he's told the hotel about his
allergies and has asked for an allergen-free meal during the flight.*

**Q   My supermarket doesn't have a 'free-from' list available yet.
Where else can I get information?**

*A   Dieticians usually have lists of foods that those with specific food allergies
should avoid. These include foods that contain specific and different types
of ingredients, which is very useful if the person with the food allergy has
to avoid more than one thing. The internet provides this information, as do
allergy-related charities, associations and support groups.*

Q   Do people grow out of their food allergy?

*A   Some people do. It depends upon the age of the person and the food
involved. Most babies will grow out of their allergy to milk, and some
children with a proven allergy to peanuts will grow out of it. However,
adults with a food allergy, for example to peanuts or shellfish, are more
likely to have it for the rest of their lives.*

19

Anaphylaxis

Not a Russian gymnast or a James Bond villain, it's a life-threatening condition. Working your way through this idea means you really could win yourself a life-saving gold medal and not fulfil 'Goldfinger's' prophecy.

Anaphylaxis is at the extreme end of the allergy spectrum. It's frightening, there's no questioning this. Frightening for the sufferer and those around him or her.

Anaphylaxis is to allergy what parachuting on a surfboard is to extreme sports. It's life threatening, but without the pleasurable buzz. Yes, it could be a foreign spy, but is better described as a lethal assassin. The weapon can be one of a number of different innocuous substances, and when they strike, speed is of the essence.

There's nothing funny about someone's face, lips, tongue and throat swelling so much that they can't speak or breathe. The whole body can be affected, sometimes within hours of exposure to the allergen, often within just minutes. The skin may flush, hives (like nettle rash) may appear anywhere on the body, abdominal

Here's an idea for you...

Develop a crisis plan for how to handle an emergency and have a trial run of what you would do. Have this plan written out for family and friends, put it on the bulletin board at home and carry a copy in your pocket. Make sure everyone knows where you keep your adrenaline (epinephrine) and how to use it.

cramping, pain and diarrhoea may occur, the person may describe a sense of impending doom and have difficulty speaking, swallowing and breathing because everything is becoming swollen, or they may feel faint and weak because their blood pressure is falling. But don't expect all these symptoms to occur because they may not. The bottom line is that any of these symptoms needs attention, and quickly.

Certain foods (e.g. peanuts, shellfish, dairy products), latex, drugs, and insect bites and stings are the usual suspects. Restaurant and food manufacturers are now very keen to inform people about what's in their foods to protect allergic individuals from problems and to protect themselves from litigation. Any food can be responsible, but it's peanuts, tree nuts (walnuts, cashews, etc.), fish, shellfish, eggs and milk that commonly cause anaphylactic reactions, and for some people only a trace is needed to set the reaction off.

Doctors too are very keen to know whether you have any allergies to particular substances, in particular to drugs like penicillin. So if you do have an allergy, particularly a severe one, don't hesitate to tell your doctor or nurse because, you never know, it may not be logged in your medical records.

Who do you spend most time with? Hopefully it's your family and friends, so make sure they know about your allergy too. And don't forget your work colleagues. You see, prevention really is better than cure, and when they make you a surprise birthday cake, if it contains something you're allergic to it may as well be laced with poison, particularly if they don't know what to do when you start to inflate like a balloon.

OK, it's time to calm things down a little. Try IDEA 29, *It's time to take 5*, and enjoy a little relaxation.

Try another idea...

Of course, it's best to avoid the triggers if you can. But how many times have you been stung by an insect because you wanted to be? How many times have you said, 'it's OK doc, I know I'm allergic to penicillin but what the heck, give it to me anyway'? Hopefully the answer is zero, nil, nada. No one wants to suffer anaphylaxis, but it can and does happen despite someone's best efforts to avoid it.

This is where it's time to make like a Cub Scout and be prepared. Those people who are known to be at risk of suffering anaphylaxis are advised to wear a Medic-Alert talisman or similar bracelet or necklace stating their allergy, so that if they should be found unconscious it's clear what action needs taking. Those at risk are also advised to carry preloaded adrenaline (epinephrine) injection kits with them and, most importantly, to learn how to use them correctly. Those around them should also know how to use these essential injections, because you never know when you are going to need to give the injection that could save your friend's life. And while we're on the subject, knowledge of basic first aid and resuscitation is never wasted either.

'A danger foreseen is half avoided.'
THOMAS FULLER, English clergyman

Defining idea...

How did it go?

Q   Why does anaphylaxis occur?

A   *Any allergic reaction, including the most extreme form, anaphylactic shock, occurs because the body's immune system reacts inappropriately in response to the presence of a substance that it wrongly perceives as a threat. An anaphylactic reaction is caused by the sudden release of chemical substances from cells in the blood and tissues where they are stored. The release is triggered by the reaction between the allergic antibody (IgE) and the substance (allergen) causing the anaphylactic reaction. This mechanism is so sensitive that minute quantities of the allergen can cause a reaction. The released chemicals act on blood vessels to cause swelling in the mouth and elsewhere on the skin, a fall in blood pressure and breathing difficulties.*

Q   How does adrenaline work?

A   *During anaphylaxis, lung tissues swell, blood vessels leak and blood pressure drops, causing choking and collapse. Adrenaline (epinephrine) is the drug of choice for treating anaphylactic reaction. It reverses the symptoms and helps prevent further progression of the reaction by relaxing smooth muscles in the lungs to improve breathing, constricting blood vessels and stimulating the heartbeat. It also helps to stop angioedema – swelling around the face and lips caused by fluid leaking out of the blood vessels – by reversing the process that allows to the blood vessels to leak.*

Q   I'm allergic to penicillin. Does this mean that my children will be too?

A   *Contrary to popular myth, a family history of allergy to a specific drug does not mean that other people in the family will also react to the same drug.*

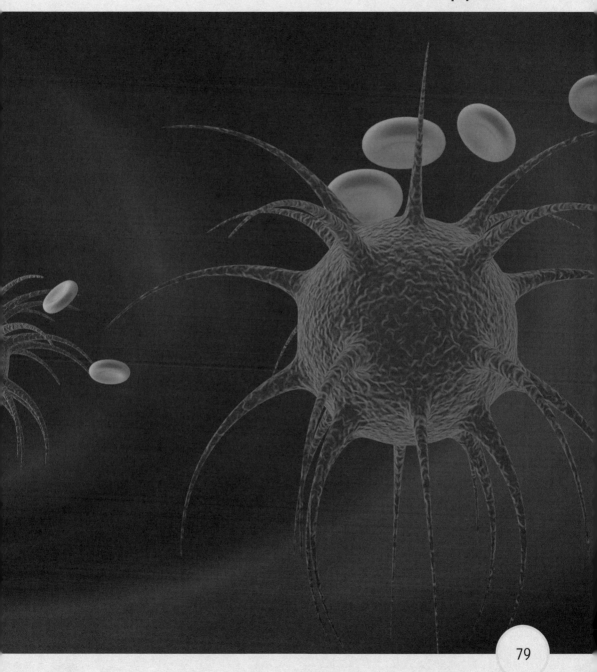

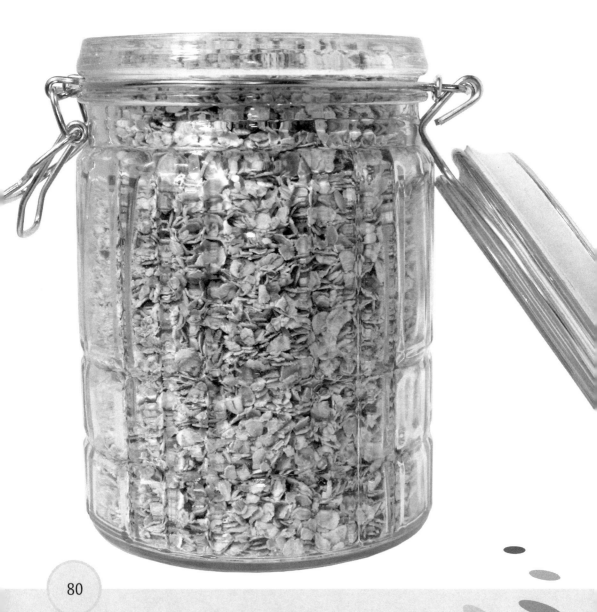

20

Getting your oats

They may be a great way to start the day, but oats are not just for the cereal bowl. Grab yourself a handful and see what else they have to offer.

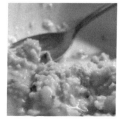

The price of cereal is a common battleground in supermarkets, the performance of wheat crops is awaited on stock exchange floors, and the sowing and getting of oats is bragged about in men's locker rooms.

The outcome of these exchanges is often some warmth and redness of the skin. It may be the warm glow of success, the displeasure, frustration or disbelief at losing the argument or the deal, or having the reality of your sexual exploits uncovered that heats the situation to boiling point and turns your cheeks red. Whether it's an emotional or physical trigger that gets under the skin, if you suffer from eczema it may not become just red and warm. It may become hot, uncomfortable and itchy, and will drive you crazy. But you can overcome this and get a soothing glow of relief somewhat akin to post-coital satisfaction. How? By getting your oats...wait for it...and rubbing them onto your irritated skin.

Here's an idea for you... **Wrap a handful of oats tightly in a muslin square, tie it firmly and put this in your bath. Then lie back in the bath and let the oatmeal get to work on you. Doing this, you'll find that your skin is soothed and less likely to become dry and itchy.**

I expect that reading this briefly conjured up images of feeding baby, or of respected pillars of society taking porridge baths for charity. It could have been worse – it could have been baked beans. But there's more to the external application of oats than raising money.

For centuries oats have been cultivated and used to aid good health. To begin with, they are rich in fibre, which helps to keep the bowel working reliably. The fibre can also help to reduce harmful levels of cholesterol, in particular damaging levels of bad cholesterol (that's low-density lipoprotein or LDL-cholesterol to those in the know), and so helps to protect the heart and circulation. Oats may also help to maintain healthy blood sugar levels. In fact, some researchers believe that people first discovered the skin-soothing effects of oatmeal nearly 4,000 years ago.

When the grain is milled, oatmeal and oatbran are produced. It's the oatmeal, the ground grain, that has a high silica content, which is used for skin problems such as eczema because it's a very good emollient. As you probably know, emollients are great for moisturising skin to prevent dryness, cracking and itching. They thus remove or reduce the temptation to scratch, and thereby prevent the further damage that is sure to happen if you succumb. Skin care manufacturers have cottoned onto this and have made products that contain oatmeal. Commercially prepared creams that can be rubbed onto the skin and bath additives containing finely ground oatmeal – known as colloidal oatmeal since it has been ground to a fine powder that will remain suspended in water – that disperse well in warm water make it easy to reap the benefits, whether the skin being soothed is irritated by eczema, sunburn, chickenpox or shingles. If you prefer a more traditional approach, a cool oatmeal compress can be placed onto the area affected to bring relief. Moreover, there's yet another use for oatmeal with regard to skin health. It can be used as a soap substitute, which is very useful since many commercial soaps remove the skin's protective oils and dry it out, which can cause it to become itchy. How do you use the oatmeal as soap? Just tie some colloidal oatmeal in a handkerchief, give it a good dunking and squeeze out any excess water. Then simply use it just as you would use your normal washcloth.

Oats – a simple food that can play such great role in helping to maintain overall health and well-being, particularly the health of the largest organ of the body, the skin. At the first inkling of this idea I suspect you were laughing at the thought of getting your oats. Now I hope you're still laughing, but for an entirely different reason.

Now you've found a great way to soothe your skin, take a look at IDEA 6, _And so to bed_, to see how to soothe your nighttime too.

Try another idea…

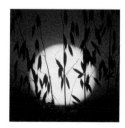

'Once we sowed wild oats, now we cook them in the microwave.'
IRENA CHALMERS, Anglo-American wit, author, teacher

Defining idea…

How did it go?

Q   Making my own 'bouquet bathi' is a bit time consuming. Are there any alternatives?

A   *Try some of the ready-made products that contain ground oatmeal, such as bath additives, which are available from the pharmacist or health store. These can be added to bath water just as you would add anything else to the bath (except, of course, your rubber duck).*

Q   I shower, and don't actually have a bath. What can I do?

A   *You can hang the muslin bag under the showerhead so the water runs through it and onto your body. This should provide you with similar benefits. If you don't have any muslin handy, then you can use a nylon stocking instead. If it's not yours, then ask permission to use it first or you'll end up with skin that is sorer than it was to start with. Alternatively you can simply use the bag of oats like a sponge and squeeze it as you press it onto your skin.*

Q   Do I still need to moisturise my skin after having a bath or shower?

A   *It's a good idea to moisturise your skin afterwards with your usual emollient cream since the process of towelling yourself dry can cause the skin to become a little dry or irritated. Oatmeal-containing creams are now readily available in stores and can help to keep your skin healthy and protected. Remember to dry yourself gently if your skin is dry or irritated. Patting the skin dry rather than rubbing it will avoid further irritation.*

21

Getting creamed

**Moisturise, moisturise, and then moisturise it some more.
This is the key to keeping skin healthy. But what should
you use and how can you avoid ending up in a sticky
mess?**

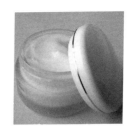

Whether it's dry skin, itchy skin or a
scorching red rash, giving the skin a gentle rub
with some cream will overcome most irritations
quickly and easily.

You've had dry skin at some time in your life. Everybody has. Perhaps you've spent
too much time in the sun, or it's the morning after the night before, or one of the
older members of your family – I'm not mentioning any names, but you know who
you are, grandad – has turned the central heating up in an attempt to convert the
living room into an oven. The skin loses its usual soft texture and feels rough. It
may feel a bit sensitive and uncomfortable too, or downright itchy. It gets like this
because it doesn't have enough natural oil to maintain the protective barrier that
should be there. No protective barrier means the skin loses moisture through

Here's an idea for you...

It's all very well having a large pot of emollient in the bathroom, but if you get itchy at work or need to travel, carrying a pot the size of a grapefruit around isn't practical. So here's the solution. Put some into a small pot that you can keep in your handbag or brief-case. This way, whenever you need to moisturise you'll always have some emollient to hand.

evaporation. Loss of moisture means the skin becomes drier and less supple. This isn't exactly nuclear physics, but the situation still needs to be reversed, and this can be done by moisturising.

Did you know that the skin is the largest organ in the body? Now there's a fact to astound and amaze your friends with. It's a fantastic piece of kit that protects bodies of all shapes and sizes. It's waterproof, too, and helps to regulate body temperature. And that's not all: when it's exposed to a little sunlight it manufactures vitamin D. So it needs looking after.

Those with skin conditions such as eczema or other skin allergies, and those who spend long periods of time in very cold or very hot weather, will have had plenty of experience of dry skin and what it feels like. They'll know how important it is to moisturise, moisturise and moisturise some more. So even though you may not want to get creamed, be it on the sports-field, in the office or anywhere else for that matter, spare a thought for your skin, which is desperate to get creamed and will love you for it.

Moisturising, or emollient therapy, to give it its correct name, is what is essential. Emollients come in cream, ointment and liquid forms (which are added to the bath), and supplement the skin's own natural oils, helping to prevent further water loss. By doing this they restore the skin's barrier function and protect it from further drying. They are also brilliant for soothing skin and relieving itching. So when you feel the need for a good scratch, don't. Rub in some emollient instead. Resist tearing at your skin with your fingernails since, although this may bring temporary relief, it will create further problems by releasing histamine, which in turn causes more itching. Scratching also causes breaks in the skin, enabling other skin irritants to enter.

Now here's the trick. When rubbing the emollient into the skin, whether it's a handful of cream or ointment you've scooped out of the pot or squeezed from a tube, gently rub it in using the pads of your fingertips, not your nails. This way you'll relieve the irritation but not light the fuse of a further itch attack. And apply it in the direction of the hairs to avoid blocking pores and hair follicles.

Now that you've discovered the benefits of moisturising, try IDEA 20, *Getting your oats*, to see how a handful of these can do you even more good than you thought.

Try another idea...

'**Have you ever been hurt and the place tries to heal a bit, and you just pull the scar off it over and over again?**'
ROSA PARKS, American civil rights activist

Defining idea...

And use plenty of it too. Be ebullient with the emollient. A great way of encouraging this behaviour is to always buy large pots of it – the more industrial the size the better. The smaller sizes may be more decorative or aesthetically pleasing, but they'll have you running to the shops every few days or using less and less as you try to eke it out. No – large pots or tubes are what you need, so you can scoop out a handful and get rubbing in earnest.

How did it go?

Q   Even when I use soaps and shower gels that are supposed to be kind to my skin it still feels very dry, even with moisturising. Do I just have to accept this?

A   *No, you don't. Many soaps and shower gels, even those marketed as beneficial for dry skin, may in fact remove the skin's protective oils, leaving it at risk of becoming dry. Try using an emollient that can also be used as a soap substitute as well as a moisturiser. This way, protective skin oils will remain trapped in the skin, reducing the chances of your skin becoming dry and irritated.*

Q   It's difficult reaching some parts of my body. What can I do?

A   *Ask a friend or your partner to apply the cream for you. Another idea is to use an emollient liquid that can be added to bath water so you actually bathe in it.*

Q **I don't want to ask anyone else to apply the cream as I'm a bit embarrassed, and I don't have a bath, only a shower. What do you suggest?**

A *Get a back-scratcher, or even a wooden spoon will do. Wrap a cloth around it and dip the cloth in the emollient cream, then apply the cream to the parts you couldn't reach with your hands.*

Q **My children hate having cream put on them. Any tips?**

A *Let them cream themselves. Give them a handful of cream to rub into their skin at the same time as you do it. They'll then see it as a fun game rather than a punishing medical treatment.*

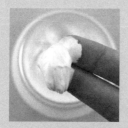
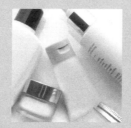
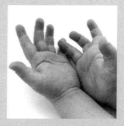

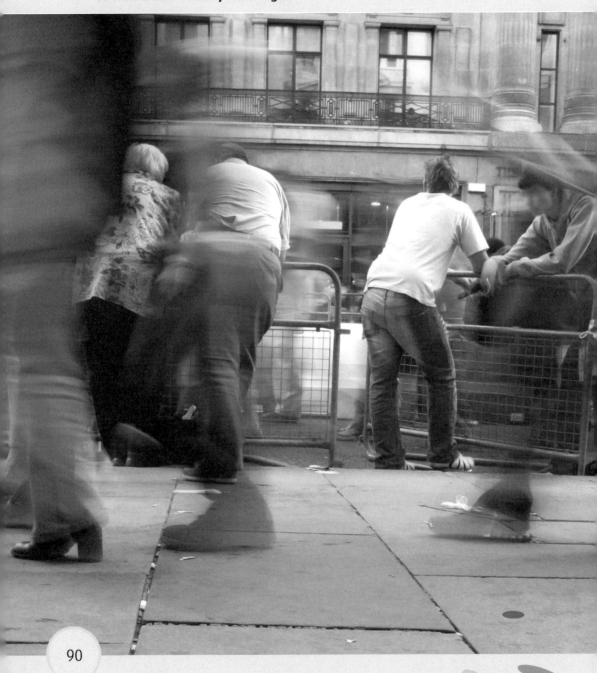

22

Risky business

Pets, pollen, poisons and poo. Let's take a look at the allergy triggers and how to be prepared if they come your way.

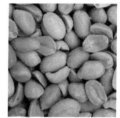

Walking down the street we watch for other people so we don't bump into them. Crossing the road, we look both ways so a passing juggernaut doesn't flatten us.

Making sure we avoid the things that may cause trouble makes life easier and more enjoyable. Often it's not the cause of the problem that's actually the problem, it's the knock-on effects. If you get stuck in a traffic jam, the problem is that you'll now be late for your meeting. If you step in something the dog's owner couldn't be bothered to pick up, you now have the unpleasant task of cleaning your shoe.

It's the same with allergy-triggering substances, or allergens. These are harmless for most people and certainly show no ill-intent, but for those who are allergic, contact with them causes all kinds of miserable problems. Pollen, for example, just wants to be left alone to do its job, but tends to spread itself about a bit in the process. The proteins in cat saliva find themselves on a journey from the cat's mouth to its fur as an essential part of the fur-cleansing process, but they can continue onto the living

Here's an idea for you...

Put together an allergy kit. To begin with this should include a check-list of what you are allergic to, what symptoms you get, ways of reducing your exposure to the allergy-triggering substance and what treatments you need. With this list keep the items you need to reduce your exposure, for example sunglasses, and the treatments you use. Check it regularly to make sure it is always complete.

room sofa and from there onto the first person who sits down. All it should need is a little brushing to remove it, but if someone is allergic to it, the ramifications can be more serious.

Whenever I find myself walking along a beach with another member of my family, at some point one of us will smile and say, 'remember when that seagull dumped on...?' We all have stories like this to tell, the details of which should remain in the family to spare the person's blushes. The seagull responsible for creating this tale must have had advanced heat-seeking technology on board, or to be more precise a breast-seeking guidance system, to have hit the target so accurately from such a distance. Then again, it could have just been male. But the member of my family who was the target for this attack was always prepared for the unexpected and in a flash a handful of tissues had wiped away the problem.

The most extreme solution to avoiding allergy triggers is to live in isolation in an environment of pure sterility. For most people, however, this is not only completely impractical – it's unnecessary. It wouldn't be much fun either. So you do your best to avoid whatever it is that lights your touch-paper, and that means some careful planning and a little preparation. Don't panic, over time it will become routine, but for this to happen you have to get into the swing of doing it.

Let's say that you're allergic to cats and are going to visit some friends. Arrangements are all made, you'll be there at 7 p.m. for dinner, and the wine is chilling nicely in the fridge. When you arrive you find that your friends have a surprise addition to their family – a pretty little kitten. If you're lucky, and prepared, then you'll have your allergy kit with you, which may include tissues, antihistamines, some eye drops and nasal spray, depending on how you react. If not, then that's probably your evening out ruined.

These risk factors may have got you a little wired, so try IDEA 9, *Chemical attack*, to formulate a strategy to keep yourself out of harm's way.

Try another idea...

But you could have avoided this. If your friends had known about your allergy – if you had told them – then you could have arranged to go out and eat instead, or they could have set up dinner in a room where the kitten isn't allowed. Basically, you could have reduced your exposure to the allergy trigger. Food manufacturers and restaurants are helping with this more and more. They put warnings on food and menus about whether the food contains nuts, for example, since many people are allergic to these. In the future we are likely to see more such warnings as the number of people with allergies increases, but until that time comes it's a good idea to be proactive and let people know that you have an allergy so they too can be prepared.

'*Let us not look back in anger, nor forward in fear, but around in awareness.*'
JAMES THURBER

Defining idea...

How did
it go?

Q **I have hayfever but love to garden. I want to be able to at least sit in my garden during the summertime. How can I avoid suffering?**

A *Start by using eye drops and nasal sprays to help prevent the allergy symptoms developing before you go into your garden. Ask your doctor or pharmacist about which ones would be suitable for you. Wear sunglasses and possibly a mask to stop pollen getting into your eyes and nose. Those who are allergic to grass pollen sometimes choose to lose some, or all, of their lawn and replace it with hard landscaping. It's also a good idea to have colourful and scented flowers that are pollinated by insects rather than wind-pollinated plants, as this will reduce your pollen exposure. Beware flowers with strong scents, though, since these can irritate those with hayfever.*

Q **If I'm going somewhere where I know I may run into allergy problems I take my kit, but every now and then I get caught out because my friend changes the plans. What should I do?**

A *You should really carry your kit with you wherever you go. People with severe allergies are always advised to do this because a chance encounter could be serious. It pays to expect the unexpected. Another good idea is to make sure that friends know what you are allergic to so that they can always have suitable over-the-counter medicines to hand should you forget yours. If you supply them yourself you know they'll be suitable. If you give your friends a list of places and things you need to avoid, they can plan accordingly.*

23

Ooh, that's gonna cost you

The cost of some treatments can cause a sharp inhalation of breath, but you don't need to get an emergency plumber and your chequebook to unblock your nose. Here are some ideas that are not to be sniffed at.

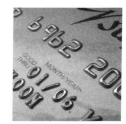

If you've ever tried talking with a blocked nose, you know that you sound ridiculous. Try eating with a blocked nose, or kissing someone. Now that's not easy.

It's a marvellous thing, the nose, and is one of our most distinctive facial, and indeed bodily, features. Ask Pinocchio, Barbra Streisand or Barry Manilow and they'll probably tell you how their nose has seen them through the good times and the bad times. In fact, they'll probably sing this for you, if you pay them enough. It's not only a person's identity that can be revealed by their nose; their cultural heritage can be too. The prominent angular Roman nose, the small rounded Oriental nose, the aristocratic French nose, ideal for smelling fine wines and perfumes. The nose can also be a source of entertainment. Think, for example, of a circus clown's big red hooter. But a congested nose is no fun at all, so here's how to unblock it.

Here's an idea for you...

To drain your sinuses once you've practised steam inhalation, try the following. For the sinuses above the eyes, sit upright for several minutes; for those between the eyes and nose, lie down on your back for several minutes; and to clear the sinuses below the eyes, lie on your opposite side to the sinus you want to drain: so, for example, to drain the left one lie on your right side for a few minutes.

Blowing the nose is the simplest option, but blowing too hard may make matters worse by sending mucus back up into the nose and sinuses, making it even more difficult to clear. Moreover, when you blow the nose too hard there's a good chance that the lining of the nasal passages will become irritated, and this irritation, in turn, will trigger the production of more mucus. It's a vicious, albeit well lubricated, circle. Since every day the nose makes an average of one litre of mucus (thankfully not all at the same time), and it makes even more when you have an allergy or a cold, any additional mucus is certainly unwelcome. So blow gently and leave the foghorn impression to the clown.

Having a blocked nose can be embarrassing. For a start, you can't breathe properly, you can't taste anything and you can't speak properly because you're totally blocked up with thick mucus that you just can't shift. Perversely, despite being totally blocked, it continually runs like a tap. You've three alternatives. You can let it drip, which makes a mess and doesn't go down well at dinner parties or formal civic receptions; you can try blowing it into a handkerchief or tissue, which could get you expelled from the cinema or theatre and makes your nose glow in the dark; or you could sniff. And how popular does that make you in the office or on a train?

Let's sniff out a few more solutions that you can put into practice calmly and easily. Taking a piece of tissue paper and gently dabbing the inside of the nose will soak up any running liquid – you know, the kind that seems to sit there trying to make it's mind up whether to take the plunge or just hang around. Sneezing is another good way of clearing the nose. It's a natural body reflex that removes unwanted stuff from the inside the nose that's causing irritation, for example dust or dirt. [Warning: if you're squeamish you may want to skip the rest of this paragraph.] Little suckers can be purchased to suck out the mucus from the nostrils, it's useful to try and loosen and soften the mucus first with steam inhalation, though, otherwise you may irritate the nose even more, or it may not only be the offending mucus that the sucker removes.

If all this mucus has got your eyes running too, sprint to IDEA 24, *Bright eyes*, and find out how to stem the flow.

Try another idea...

Just because you're all blocked up doesn't mean you have to miss out on the kissing too. OK, it may not be possible, or kind, to do it the French way, but you can always follow the Eskimos and rub noses.

'Knowing is not enough, you must apply; willing is not enough, you must do.'
BRUCE LEE

Defining idea...

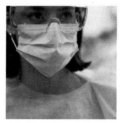
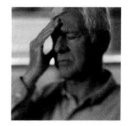

How did
it go?

Q   What about using decongestant medication?

A   *Decongestant nasal drops, sprays and tablets work by constricting blood vessels in the nose and sinuses, thereby reducing inflammation. They work quickly to dry up excess secretions and provide fast, effective relief from a blocked or runny nose. A note of caution, though: some of these should only be used for a few days, as using them for more than a week can result in rebound nasal congestion which can make the blocked nose worse. If in doubt, read the label.*

Q   Sneezing is a pretty good way of clearing the nose, but you can't sneeze to order can you?

A   *Well, yes you can. If you irritate your nose, then you will sneeze. As a child you must have tried to make someone sneeze by tickling their nose with a feather or a hair. Well, it's the same principle. Bearing in mind that often you just can't find a feather when you want one, try gently tickling the inside of the nose with a wisp of cotton wool. This should produce a helpful ahh-choo.*

Q   I was told to put saline nose drops into my nose. Is there anything else I can use instead of a dropper?

A   *Try using a cotton wool ball. Soak this in the saline solution and then let the saline gently drip into the nose. Sometimes it's easier to do this lying down because it can take time for the drops to leave the cotton wool.*

24

Bright eyes

When your eyes are burning like fire you need something to soothe them quickly. Here are some ideas for you to keep in your sights.

Whether you're happily out and about enjoying yourself or taking a few minutes to relax and unwind, if something gets into your eye that shouldn't be there it's unpleasant.

Your eyes are often the first thing people notice about you and are said to be the windows on the soul. Sparkling eyes are an indication of good health. Red, watering, itchy eyes that are gummed up with mucus are saying something completely opposite. Whether it's because of the swelling, the water or your scratching hands being in the way, you can't see clearly and you're in desperate need of some relief.

Whatever the allergy trigger is – pollen, house dust mite dung, animal dander or perfume – once it gets up your nose and into your eyes it sparks the release of chemicals. Even eye drops, contact lenses and contact-lens solutions may be responsible for triggering an upset. These chemicals initiate a chain reaction, and

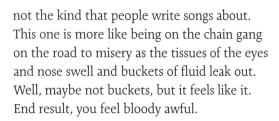

A cold compress is an excellent and practical reliever. Make your own from cotton pads soaked in rosewater, witch-hazel or cold camomile tea. In fact, make yourself a relaxing cup of camomile herbal tea and reuse the cooled teabag as an eye compress. Cucumber slices are an old favourite. A 20 minute session will help you see the world through happier eyes.

not the kind that people write songs about. This one is more like being on the chain gang on the road to misery as the tissues of the eyes and nose swell and buckets of fluid leak out. Well, maybe not buckets, but it feels like it. End result, you feel bloody awful.

For most people, it's the itching that's the most frustrating and irritating symptom. You can hide your red eyes from everyone else's gaze by wearing shades, and even the watering can be absorbed onto a tissue. But the itching, that's what drives people crazy and gets in the way of their regular, everyday activities.

You know you shouldn't, but they're crying out to be rubbed, and so rub them you do. This may make your eyes feel a whole lot better and clear the blurred vision, but this is only a temporary respite. It's just like driving down the motorway in a rainstorm: the windscreen wipers briefly give you a clear view of the road ahead, but as soon as they have passed the screen is covered again. But why does rubbing only make them worse?

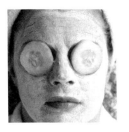

It seems logical that, once the irritating culprit has done it's dirty deed and the chemicals that cause the problem have been used up, the itching and the watering should finish. However, where the eyes are concerned, this is not the case. (In this regard, they are just like mosquito bites.) Rubbing your eyes can have the same effect as the allergy trigger that got into your eyes in the first place: it causes more of the chemicals, for example histamine, to be released. However, it does this mechanically rather than chemically, as the act of rubbing in effect bursts the chemical-containing cells, releasing the chemicals and allowing them to kick into action. So here's the stinger: when it comes to the eyes, if you've got an itch don't scratch it. You need to find relief some other way.

You've tried some soothing ideas for sore eyes; now try IDEA 30, *Let's chill*, and see how to take the heat out of other swollen body parts.

Try another idea...

A cold compress, using a face cloth soaked in cold water, is a great idea because it's soothing and, being cold, will stabilise the cells that contain those triggering chemicals and prevent more of them escaping. Cold also helps to relieve inflammation. Anti-allergy eye drops are also very good at helping to relieve symptoms, and if someone suffers on a regular basis, using them each day can help to prevent the symptoms too.

So here's the golden rule. At all times, fingers should be kept out of eyes. No ifs, no buts. You wouldn't poke yourself in the eye, would you? No. So don't rub or scratch them either.

'When the itch is inside the boot, scratching outside provides little consolation.'
CHINESE PROVERB

Defining idea...

How did it go?

Q   I've heard that eyebright is good for eyes. What is it?

A   *Eyebright (or Euphrasia officinalis, to use its official name) is a herb that helps to keep the eyes bright and maintain eye health. More specifically, its anti-inflammatory properties help to ease congestion and relieve uncomfortable inflammation, stinging and weeping. To make a compress, place a teaspoonful of the dried herb in half a litre (1 pint) of water and boil for 10 minutes, let it cool then soak some cotton wool, muslin or gauze in the lukewarm liquid, wring out slightly and place over the eyes.*

Q   Can eyewash help?

A   *Yes, bathing the eyes can be very soothing and also helps to remove mucus and allergy-triggering material (allergens) such as pollen from the eye. A variety of preparations are available from the pharmacist to bathe or irrigate the eyes. Artificial tears can help too since they can dilute and remove the allergens from the eyes.*

Q   Does environment play a part? I find that when I'm at the coast my eyes are not so bad.

A   *Many factors, including activity, temperature and humidity, can affect how often and how badly someone suffers allergic eye symptoms. Hot and dry weather usually makes things worse, whereas cooler temperatures seem to alleviate the symptoms, which may explain why you feel better near the coast. Pollen in particular is more easily dispersed in coastal areas because sea breezes blow it inland, and it's less likely to be produced in cooler climates. The sea air is also beneficial, especially in easing nasal allergic symptoms.*

25

A tissue, a tissue

The world record for the longest sneezing bout is 978 days, but this isn't a record you want to beat. Try this idea to stop the sneezes.

First comes the tickle, next the build-up, and before you know it it's Ah, Ahh, Ahhh – Choo! And if you're not careful, you'll be stuck in repeat mode.

The urge to sneeze comes out of the blue and is difficult to avoid. And it often seems to happen when you are in awkward places, like museums or the theatre, and at inconvenient times, like during interviews or when making love. Yes, even then. Some sex therapists use the sneeze to explain to people about the sensation of orgasm. OK, I suppose they are similar: there's the build up, the point of no return and the inevitable relief that may be accompanied by a soft 'oo' or an earth-moving roar. Both are apparently pleasurable and end with a feeling of relief and well-being, though I know which one I'd choose. Multiple orgasms are a pleasure to strive for, but multiple sneezing is simply a pain – so how can you stop it?

If a sneeze comes upon you at an inconvenient moment – say, you're out of tissues or out at the theatre – stifle it in the following way. At the onset of the urge to sneeze, push your index finger into the dimple above your upper lip. Keep applying pressure until the urge simply goes away.

Sneezing, also called sternutation, is a bodily reflex that removes an irritation from your nose. It's a sudden, forceful, involuntary burst of air through the nose and mouth that involves a very complex process. When the inside of your nose becomes irritated a message is sent to the sneeze centre in the brain, which in turn sends a message to all the muscles involved in sneezing – abdominal, chest, diaphragm, throat and eyelid muscles – to make sure that they work as a team and in the right order to eject the irritation from your nose.

It's not just snotty jobsworths getting up your nose that can irritate you: pretty much anything that gets up there can flick the switch of the sneeze mechanism. Viral infections that cause coughs and colds, dust, cold air, even steroid nasal spray treatment can result in sneezing. For those with allergies, pollen, house dust mite dung and animal dander are the common culprits. Then there's certain (illegal) recreational substances and, of course, pepper – remember buying sneezing powder from the joke shop? Even tweezing eyebrows, combing your hair or eating too much can trigger sneezing. Keeping out of the way of the offending substance, or simply stopping what you're doing, means the sneezing should disappear.

Have a think about your sternutatory habits. It's important to consider those around you when you sneeze. For one thing, you don't want to burst their eardrums. And for another, you don't want to cover them in snot, which is easily done, since sneezing can send it five feet or more. Not only could you be banned from where you are for doing this, it could also get you banned from driving. How? Well, the discharge when you sneeze travels at speeds up to, and sometimes slightly over, 100 mph. More seriously though, when we sneeze our eyes close as part of the automatic response and during that minuscule period of time you could have driven into someone or something. Sneezing is a very effective way of spreading germs too when you have a cough or a cold – one sneeze can spray 10 million germs, which is why you should cover your mouth and nose, preferably with a tissue that can be discarded afterwards. Failing this, wash your hands so you don't leave germs on telephones, door handles, etc. that other people may come into contact with.

So now you can stop a sneeze in its tracks. Try IDEA 1, *Going into overdrive*, to get to the root of allergies and what you can do about them.

Try another idea...

So next time you feel the need to sneeze, and your eyes automatically close to prevent getting back spray, think carefully about whether you really want to splatter your loved one with snot. Because if you do it's not just a wet nose you'll be left with, the thump you get may leave it considerably bruised too.

'Success is to be measured not so much by the position that one has reached in life as by the obstacles which he has overcome.'
BOOKER T. WASHINGTON, educator and black leader

Defining idea...

How did
it go?

Q   What's the best way of preventing sneezing if you have allergies?

A   *Avoiding exposure to the offending allergen is the most effective way. This may mean using an air filtration unit in the home, keeping pets outside or staying indoors on days when the pollen count is high, for example. When this isn't enough or is not practical, then using allergy treatments such as antihistamines or steroidal nasal sprays helps.*

Q   I often sneeze when I go outside into the sunshine. Is this normal?

A   *Most people have some sensitivity to light that can trigger a sneeze. Around one in four people suffer with 'sun sneezing' or the 'ACHOO syndrome', where sudden exposure to bright light triggers sneezing. Bright light can sometimes help with sneezing too. If a sneeze gets stuck – you know, when you feel you want to sneeze but it just won't come – briefly looking at a bright light (not into the sun) can bring out the sneeze.*

Q   After a sneeze, people often say, 'God bless you!' Why?

A   *One theory is that it started as a blessing by Pope Gregory I the Great (540–604 AD) during the plague of 590 AD. When someone sneezed, they were immediately blessed ('God bless you!') in the hope that they would not subsequently develop the plague. Another is that in the Middle Ages people believed that sneezing blew your soul out from within your body, making it fair game for the devil to take. However, if someone said 'God Bless You' your soul would be returned to the sanctuary of your body.*

26

Rubber rising

If the touch of rubber raises your hackles rather than your pulse, or anywhere else for that matter, here's an idea to rub away the problem.

Rubber comes in all shapes and sizes and colours. Gloves and wetsuits provide necessary protection when we need it. Other items of rubber bring pleasure and protection when we want it.

Sadly it's those rubber products we come into contact with most often, and for some may well bring the most pleasure, which most often cause reactions. So do you need to miss out? No, you don't – and here's how.

Allergy to the latex in rubber comes in two distinct forms. Natural proteins in latex cause the immediate type of reaction, where hives or nettle rash, itching, redness, swelling, sneezing, wheezing or, rarely, life-threatening anaphylaxis occurs within seconds of contact. Additives called rubber accelerators are responsible for the

Here's an idea for you...

Keep cotton gloves around your home, in your car, your office, and in your handbag or briefcase too. Wear them around the house, under waterproof gloves if you're doing wet jobs and under any latex gloves that you have to wear. For those with contact hand dermatitis, doing this will protect the hands from further irritation.

delayed type that usually takes around 48 hours to kick in (but can take less) and causes skin irritation, known as contact dermatitis, at or around the point of contact. It's not only rubber that can cause contact dermatitis, though. You may have heard older women talking about their suspenders and how the metal components would leave a red mark. This was not caused by them pressing too hard on the skin, or by frenzied twanging during moments of friskiness. It was actually caused by sensitivity to nickel, which, even though the suspender belt may be lost in the undergarments of time, still exists today. Nowadays, however, it's more likely to be the studs in denim jeans or body-piercings that cause the red, itchy and irritating marks of contact dermatitis.

Bouncing back to rubber, it's thought that the increased use of latex gloves as a result of infection precaution policies in health care facilities, and changes in processes used to manufacture latex products, are behind the increase in allergy to proteins in natural rubber latex. As with so many things, progress benefits on the one hand, whilst it quite literally may cause additional problems on the other hand. And to combat these new challenges have come unpowdered, low-allergen gloves and continuous research into developing latex products containing less latex allergen. Although most often it's the hands that are affected, it can occur anywhere on the body where rubber gets into contact. So when he, or she, says that using a condom is irritating, it may be true in more ways than one.

During the run-up to my finals, I was warned by a hospital consultant – who, in the interest of preventing any inflammation, shall remain nameless but who was feared by many – to remember to use the little sachet of talcum powder found with the examination gloves should I find myself in front of him during my final exams. The reason behind his advice was that my palms would be so sweaty that it would be impossible for me to get the gloves on. And it's true, trying to put on a pair of rubber gloves with sweaty palms and without powder is nigh-on impossible.

Now that you've firmly grasped how to avoid rubber-related problems, try IDEA 21, *Getting creamed*, to find out how a little bit of cream can help control allergies.

Try another idea...

To overcome this, powdered latex gloves can be used. Unfortunately, with powdered gloves the latex allergens become airborne, making it easy for them to be inhaled or to come into contact with the nose or eyes and subsequently trigger symptoms. This is exactly why the main problem with latex allergy is with powdered gloves, since these release an estimated 15,000 times more allergy-triggering substances into the air than unpowdered ones. Like latex gloves made without additional chemicals, unpowdered gloves and synthetic ones, for example vinyl gloves, are often better to use.

'There's a new medical crisis. Doctors are reporting that many men are having allergic reactions to latex condoms. They say they cause severe swelling. So what's the problem?'
PHYLLIS DILLER, actress and comedian

Defining idea...

109

My final exam was indeed in front of the same consultant, and, remembering his words, I dutifully opened the sachet. Like the allergens from latex gloves, the sachet contents flew into the air and all over his designer suit. Well, he'd omitted to warn me about controlling the anxiety-fuelled shaking hands I was experiencing, so I don't think I was completely to blame for his consequent irritation!

How did it go?

Q I have a latex rubber allergy and recently I've found that I'm reacting to some foods too. Why?

A   *This sounds like cross-reactivity. Some of the allergenic proteins found in latex may also be found in bananas, kiwi fruit, avocados and chestnuts. If you're allergic to latex you may also react to these foods too. It's because of an enzyme called chitinase, which in nature protects plants from undesirable insects. The rubber tree's sap is packed with chitinase, and the others possess it too.*

Q What about latex paint? If you have latex rubber allergy do you need to avoid this?

A   *Latex paints don't contain natural rubber latex so usually don't tend to cause problems.*

Q   Which occupations are most risky for developing latex allergy?

A   *Anyone who has to wear latex rubber gloves during their work may be at risk. Hospital workers have traditionally been the most commonly affected, although with increased concern about hygiene and infection control in other professions it may not be long before these catch up.*

Q   I need to wash my hands regularly in my work and it doesn't help my skin at all. Any tips please?

A   *Try using an emollient cream instead of soap. It can cleanse the hands and skin just as well, but also helps the skin to retain its protective oils. And if possible, wash your hands less frequently.*

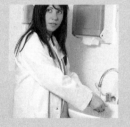 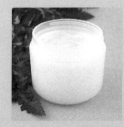 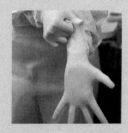

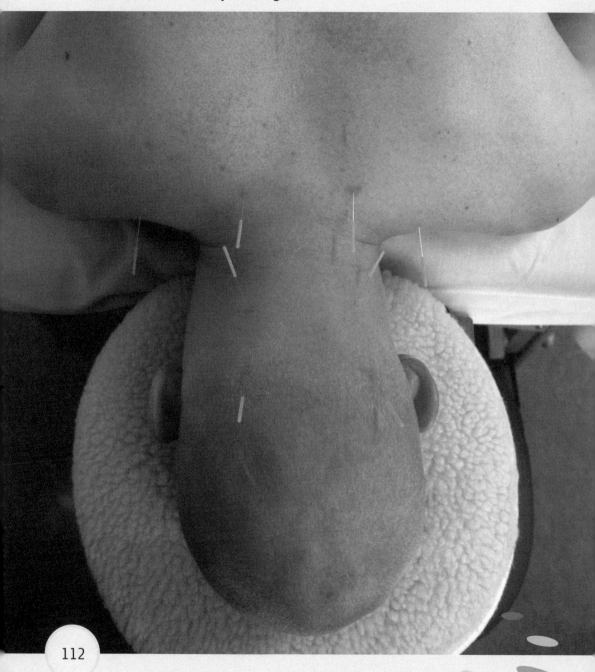

27

Sticking the needle in

A little prick with a needle, that's what the doctor said. Then came another, and another. How acupuncture can help to overcome the problems of allergy.

You're going to stick that where? Well please be gentle when you do it. Oh, you've done it already. Good heavens, I didn't feel a thing.

The term acupuncture comes from the Greek *acus* (needle) and *punctura* (puncture). It literally means 'to prick with a needle' – so if you're ever in Greece on a moped and some prick with a needle forces you off the road and bursts your tyres, you'll know what to call him. Acupuncture and acupressure can also help take the sting out of allergies too.

It's not just bean-munching hippies who support the benefits of acupuncture. Modern-day science, through properly performed scientific studies, has shown how acupuncture can help to treat the symptoms of many different conditions. The pain of arthritis, for example, responds well, and the relief from and prevention of the symptoms of allergy can also be achieved by the pointed application of needles.

Here's an idea for you...

With your palm facing down and using your other thumb, press in the 'V' between your index finger and thumb. This is an antihistamine point. Place direct pressure underneath the bone that attaches to your index finger and hold your thumb there firmly for one minute whilst breathing deeply. Repeat on your other hand. A word of warning – don't do this if you're pregnant as it can cause premature contractions of the uterus.

Studies have demonstrated that people receiving real acupuncture had fewer allergy symptoms and more allergy-free days than those receiving pretend, or sham, acupuncture. What appeals to many people who suffer with allergies is that having regular acupuncture treatments means they don't have to take so much medication. Moreover, acupuncture can be used safely by both adults and children.

Even though it's only recently that modern medicine has started to embrace it, acupuncture has been practised for more than 5,000 years. It was ancient Chinese soldiers who first noticed that when their opponents' arrows injured them, other illnesses they suffered from miraculously disappeared. Not a bad pay-off if the arrow caused only a minor flesh wound and your thirty-day headache disappeared. Not so great if the arrow meant you quickly left this world but without that irritating fungal toenail infection. They noticed that the vital factor was the position of the arrow wound, and so developed the philosophy of acupuncture, it's meridian channels, and the belief that restoring the body's energy (or Qi) or life force could cure disease and illness.

Of course, progress has meant that to benefit from acupuncture you no longer have to assume the role of William Tell's slightly taller son. And if you think that those who practise acupuncture are simply trying to inflict pain by legitimate means, then think about this. You've probably had a blood test, a vaccination, or an ear or other body part pierced, haven't you? It may have hurt a little, but you coped. Well acupuncture needles, being a lot finer, are much less uncomfortable when placed into your skin. In fact, unless you have a pain threshold which is so low that if someone breaks wind you scream, you probably won't feel a thing.

Whilst we're on the subject of complementary therapies, let me point you to IDEA 42, The mother of all remedies.

Try another idea...

So here's the point. Acupuncture can help overcome the misery of allergy symptoms. In fact, you don't even have to visit a Chinese practitioner to have the treatment, as many conventionally trained doctors are now trained in acupuncture techniques too.

A word of warning: where needles are concerned, it's definitely a case of don't try this at home. If you feel the need, try acupressure instead. With this, rather than inserting a needle at specific points around the body, you press those same points with your finger and gain a similar effect. And it's simple to do. In fact, you may have already done it, pressing your finger or thumb against the inside of your wrist to try and overcome travel sickness, for example. It's acupressure that those elastic wristbands with the plastic button in them are used for, again to overcome travel sickness, morning sickness or sickness resulting from a night on the town. So what are you waiting for? Whether it's pressure or a needle, why not give it a go for your allergies?

'Life opens up opportunities to you, and you either take them or you stay afraid of taking them.'
JIM CARREY

Defining idea...

Q **I get swollen eyes a lot with my allergy. What can I do?**

A   *You need to activate your Heavenly Pillar, or point B 10. This is on the ropy muscles below the base of your skull. Place your palm against the back of your neck, about 1–2 cm below the base of the skull and 1–2 cm away from your spine. Press your fingers into the neck muscles on the side of the spine and hold this for one minute. Then repeat, using your other hand to press the other side. Applying a cool compress soaked in camomile (to the eyes, not the neck) is another wonderfully effective way of relieving swollen and sore eyes.*

Q **Itchy skin is my main allergy problem. It starts at the most inconvenient times. Can acupuncture help?**

A   *Try dipping into your Crooked Pond, or point LI 11, sited on your forearm near the elbow crease. Ideally you should have your sleeves rolled up so that you can see your elbow crease, but it's not essential. First of all, bend one arm so that your forearm is across your body and your palm is down. Press your thumb into your elbow joint on top of the arm at the point where the elbow crease ends. Hold this firmly for one minute whilst breathing deeply. Then repeat on the other arm.*

Q **What about sinus congestion? Can acupressure help with this?**

A   *Without doubt. Closing your eyes, place two fingertips between your eyes and eyebrows along the bridge of your nose in line with your sinuses. Slowly massage in firm circles.*

28

Activity zone

You may think that having an allergy gives you the perfect excuse for not exercising. Well I'm afraid you need to think again, because exercise may be just what the doctor orders.

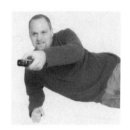

Pressing the TV remote control button, turning the car steering wheel, climbing out of bed. That's about the size of it when it comes to physical activity these days. We do 'nuffin'. At least, we don't do nearly enough.

Thirty minutes of moderately intensive exercise on at least five days of the week is what is currently recommended if you are to benefit your health. Your doctor suggests you should do more exercise, and the toned models in magazines recommend the same, though in a slightly different way. Being active on a daily basis not only helps reduce our risk of nasty killer diseases, it also helps keep our mood lifted and can keep our allergies at bay too.

Carrying too much weight increases your risk of a premature exit from this world as a result of heart disease, diabetes and some cancers. It means clothes that used to bring you pleasure stay in the wardrobe or bring tears to your eyes as you try to do

Here's an idea for you...

To benefit our health, we should aim for 10,000 steps a day. Write down how many steps you think you take during each day of the week. Then get a pedometer and see how close you were with your estimate and how close you are to the 10,000-step target. If you're already there, congratulations; now try increasing the target by 500 steps each week. If you're not quite there yet, keep at it.

them up. Moderate aerobic exercise strengthens your immune system, making it less sensitive to allergens. Exercise also helps the parts of the body affected by allergies, for example the nasal passages and lungs, to function well. Whether you prefer running, cycling, dancing or swimming, it all helps.

Mention the word exercise and it's not long before you start thinking about lycra-clad bodies in a gym. Some look great, others look like their lycra runneth over. If the thought of bodies in a gym pumping away, muscles rippling, sweat trickling down towards the base of the spine, chests heaving – sorry, got carried away there – does it for you, then great, off to the gym you go. For many, though, the term exercise is enough to send them staggering in the opposite direction in search of a bag of crisps to munch whilst surfing the TV. This means they'll be exposed to the millions of allergy-triggering house dust mites that have also made themselves at home on the couch. It also means their lungs will not get the chance to be used to the full and, since inactivity encourages obesity, breathing may become even more difficult.

But you don't have to join a gym to exercise. Start by simply going for a walk each day. Briskly is good, and ideally for about 30 minutes. If 30 minutes in one go is too difficult, break it up into shorter blocks of 15, 10 or even 5 minutes. It goes without saying that you should avoid allergy symptom triggers as best you can, so if you have hayfever, for example, don't take your walk across fields during peak pollen times.

If walking isn't your thing, do anything energetic that you enjoy. Dance to music, for example, or seek out that old exercise bike you bought so that you'd fit into your Brazilian-style beachwear but never got round to unwrapping. It's your choice.

Activity is vital for good health and helping keep allergies under control. So is not smoking, so drag yourself over to IDEA 45, *Send it packing*, because it's time to quit.

Try another idea...

I know what you are thinking: that you don't have time. If this is really true, try doing the things you do every day but in a slightly different way. Walk rather than drive to the newsagent's shop. At the supermarket park at the far side of the car park rather than as close to the entrance as you can get. When travelling to and from work get off the bus one stop earlier and walk the rest of the way; use the stairs instead of the lift; and at work, whilst waiting for the photocopying to be done, instead of leaning against the machine take a walk to see colleagues. These activities may be simple, but they all count. At home, vacuuming and other housework counts – but remember to wear a mask if you have a house dust mite allergy that makes you sneeze and bungs up your nose. Gardening counts, too. In fact, practically any activity helps.

So what are you waiting for? Go on, get active. You'll feel better in yourself as those endorphins flood your mind and body, and your allergies will be better controlled.

'Those who don't find time for exercise will have to find time for illness.'
15TH EARL OF DERBY

Defining idea...

**Q   I actually want to do some challenging physical exercise. What
would be a good one to do if I have allergies?**

A   *Swimming is a great exercise for a number of reasons. To begin with, it
doesn't put intense pressure on joints, unlike running, for example, since the
water supports the body. It's particularly good for those with asthma since it's
less likely to trigger wheezing. The moist air prevents the airways from drying
out and so it's helpful for those with a stuffy nose caused by allergic rhinitis.*

Q   Is it OK to exercise if you have asthma?

A   *Beliefs have completely turned around in recent years, and no longer are
those with asthma advised to avoid exercise and physical activity. In fact,
they're positively encouraged to exercise within their capability. Being active
promotes better lung function, and it's emotionally uplifting too. Even those
with exercise-induced asthma are encouraged to be physically active since
this still helps. Of course, you should always confirm with your doctor or
specialist that it is OK for you to do this.*

**Q   I find it difficult to motivate myself to walk or exercise regularly.
Any tips for me?**

A   *It should be reward enough that your allergy symptoms are better
controlled, but it's often very difficult to keep motivated, especially when
the rewards do not come quickly. To keep motivated, change your route or
the exercise you do, listen to music whilst doing it, or challenge yourself to
do a bit more within the 30 minutes. Doing it with a friend always helps to
maintain motivation and can be more fun too.*

29

It's time to take 5

Relaxation benefits the mind and body, so empty your mind, release the symptoms of allergy and be free...

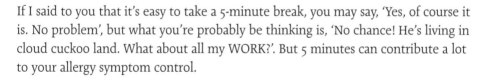

Five minutes. It's not very long, is it? Time to make a cup of coffee, time to go to the bathroom, time to overcook an egg. There's a lot you can achieve in five minutes.

If I said to you that it's easy to take a 5-minute break, you may say, 'Yes, of course it is. No problem', but what you're probably be thinking is, 'No chance! He's living in cloud cuckoo land. What about all my WORK?'. But 5 minutes can contribute a lot to your allergy symptom control.

Our increasingly stressed 24/7 environment, with longer working hours and less time to enjoy ourselves, is certainly contributing to poorer health. Maybe not always directly, but certainly by pushing us into unhealthy lifestyle behaviours. As far as allergies are concerned, being stressed doesn't help either. Everything feels worse when we are stressed, and that in turn makes the itchy eyes or itchy skin worse, and so on. When we are stressed we don't handle things so well either, so they can get on top of us and become overwhelming.

Here's an idea for you...

Next time you go and have a pee, time yourself. My guess is that it will take around 5 minutes, all in. Now, you don't feel bad about going for a pee, do you? So, take a similar break every hour just to chill out. You'll feel more relaxed throughout the day, you'll still get your work completed, and you may even find yourself with time to spare.

It's part of good stress management to take a break every now and then. During the year it's a holiday, during the week it's the weekend, during the day it's the lunch break, and during each hour it should be at least 5 minutes. If you're feeling guilty about even thinking about having a 5-minute break each hour, ask yourself why. You don't feel guilty about planning and taking a holiday, do you? Or having the weekend off? Of course not. OK, your colleagues may make you feel guilty about taking a lunch break when they work through theirs. But even though they may think this behaviour enhances their career prospects, in the long run it's likely to be damaging their health, so they may not survive to realise those career prospects anyway.

You're bound to have heard people saying that it's important to take regular breaks throughout the working day. Most people can't concentrate properly for more than 45 minutes at a time. In fact, many people can't really concentrate effectively for longer than 20 minutes. So once you pass the point where you are no longer concentrating effectively – you know when I mean, it's when you're sitting in front of the spreadsheet on your computer screen but your mind is wandering, perhaps you're thinking about doing some internet surfing, or you're playing with your pen more than you are reading the report in your hands – you may as well take a break. You're not doing anything constructive anyway, and the chances are that the only things that will happen are mistakes, which ironically will probably take longer than 5 minutes to correct.

We react negatively to the suggestion of a short break because we don't believe that 5 minutes will be just 5 minutes. We've been brainwashed into believing it'll be much longer. 'Oh, it will only take you a minute', says your boss. Well, if that's true, why doesn't she do it herself instead of taking even longer to explain it to you?

I know one person for whom the thought of a 5-minute break was a complete anathema. A colleague suggested that every time he felt his mind wandering, he take a minute or two to stretch, unwind and relax. All he did was get up and walk to the other side of the room and back, before returning to what he was doing. Before long he was in the habit of doing this automatically, without even thinking about it. The work got done, he felt better and more relaxed throughout the day, he had a healthier lifestyle and even his allergy was better controlled. So, despite what you may have initially thought, only a 5-minute break spent relaxing is long enough to do us some good.

That wasn't so bad, was it? Ready for the big one? OK. Take a deep breath, sit back and enjoy IDEA 52, *Go on, you've earned it.*

Try another idea...

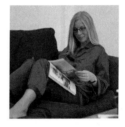

'All great achievements require time.'
MAYA ANGELOU

Defining idea...

How did
it go?

**Q   I keep forgetting to take a break because I'm so tied up with
work. How can I overcome this?**

A   *Set an alarm on your watch, clock or mobile phone to go off every hour to
remind you. Do it with a friend or colleague, since this makes it easier. Just
do whatever it takes for you to grab those valuable 5 minutes each hour.*

**Q   Most of my working day is spent in meetings. I can hardly up and
off for 5 minutes, can I?**

A   *Most people can't concentrate effectively for longer than 45 minutes, so use
this as a reason to 'take 5, everybody'. That way, everyone else will benefit,
too. Comfort breaks are acceptable, and if you take the long route you'll get
your 5-minute break. Try fixing meetings for no longer than an hour. This
way, you'll always get the opportunity to have your 5 minutes.*

**Q   Five minutes seems much too long for me. By 3 minutes I'm
getting anxious and clock-watching, waiting to get back to work.
Can't I cut my breaks short?**

A   *If taking the time is making you anxious then it's not going to be having
the desired effect. Try just taking a 1 minute break each hour for a week,
and then 2 minutes the next week and so on, so that you build up gradually
until you can comfortably enjoy the full 5 minutes. However, if fewer
minutes are really all you really need, then that's fine.*

30

Let's chill

Elvis, the Fonz, Madonna. These icons of cool knew how to keep things chilled. When allergy is in your neighbourhood you need to keep cool too. Here's how.

Kids running in and out of the garden hosepipe spray. Pouring a bottle of cold water over your head so it flows over your face and onto your body. You've done it once — so why not do it again?

I remember taking part in a stress-management seminar where the tutor asked us what we did to reduce our stress. Some said that they went out for dinner, others said that they went on holiday, I said that I liked to drive my car. All too impractical, he told us. You can't go on holiday each time your boss winds you up. How on earth could driving in a congested city be relaxing, he challenged? He had a point, but I argued that I enjoyed being in a car regardless of where I was, whilst driving I could listen to relaxing music and, unlike the other suggestions from the group, mine could be used instantly. He conceded that perhaps my idea wasn't so bad after all because what's important when you need to cool down emotionally, or physically, is

Wrap a bag of frozen vegetables in a cloth and place them on the area of your body that's sore, itchy, swollen or uncomfortable for one or two minutes. If you're going to place them on your forehead or over your eyes, wrap them in a double cloth so that it feels cool rather than cold. Frozen peas or sweetcorn are best because, being small, they adapt to the shape of your body more effectively. But even broccoli will do.

that what you use is quick, practical and easily accessible. And this is what's needed when your allergy means your eyes are burning, your nose is throbbing or your skin is tearing you apart.

Cool water fits the bill perfectly. And not only is it simple, effective, quick and accessible – it's cheap, too! Like many things in life, though, the key is how you use it.

Water in its solid form as ice is used to relieve the discomfort and pain of inflammation. One of the first things the team physio or doctor does when treating a sporting injury is to put an ice pack onto the injured area. I remember being amazed, and delighted, at how quickly the swelling went down in the joint I had injured whilst being too enthusiastic in the gym. Ice is simple and it's very effective.

Cold compresses are great if you don't have ice available. Basically it's just a cloth, for example a face cloth, soaked in cool water. There's no need to be overdramatic when you use these. You don't need a chaise longue to stretch out on, or a 1930s-style beau to calm your fevered brow. Simply soaking the compress in cooled herbal tea, such as camomile, and placing it over closed eyes will do the job of relieving sore, itchy and red eyes nicely.

Splashing some water from a running tap over your face will soon bring relief to sore eyes. You know this because you are bound to have done it at some time in your life, whether you have allergies or simply because you needed to wake yourself up. Gargling water when you have a sore or itchy throat is similarly helpful. The word eczema comes from the ancient Greek and literally means 'to boil over', and if you've got eczema you'll know that it's aptly named. If you don't have eczema, then think back to when you got sunburned having fallen asleep by the pool. Well, having eczema can feel something like this. Just allowing the water from the cold tap to flow gently over your hands and arms is very relaxing emotionally, and it's soothing for the skin too.

As you can see, keeping cool when your allergies have got you under pressure is a good idea and doesn't mean taking a cold shower or jumping into the plunge pool at the sauna either – unless, of course, that's what does it for you! It takes all sorts after all.

Cooling down a heated situation is important. Try IDEA 31, *De-stress de stress*, to learn about the best ways to achieve this.

Try another idea...

'Aaaayhh!'
THE FONZ

Defining idea...

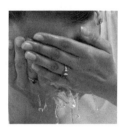

How did it go?

Q **The fridge at work doesn't have a freezer compartment so I've nowhere to keep frozen vegetables! I'm not keen to waste water either. Any ideas?**

A   *Fill a new plant water spray container with cold water, label it so others know what it is, and keep it in the fridge. Use it to spray a mist of cool water onto your face or skin. This is both refreshing and water efficient. Cool packs are available nowadays that can be instantly used and don't need to be kept refrigerated. They are often used to ease headaches too. You just remove them from their packaging, place them onto the skin and hey, presto! You feel cool again.*

Q **I spend a lot of my working day out and about. Do you have any tips for keeping cool on the move?**

A   *A mini-fan will fit into your handbag or briefcase nicely, and is both practical and easily accessible. Make sure you always have spare batteries available, though, because the Law of Sod dictates that when you need to use it the batteries will have run down.*

Q **My skin really feels like it's burning when it plays up. Sometimes my emollient creams are not that effective. Is there anything else I can do?**

A   *Try keeping your emollient cream in the fridge. It can feel wonderful and is very soothing when lightly chilled. Always make sure that it's stored safely out of children's reach and it's clear that it's not food so some unsuspecting visitor doesn't mistake it for cream cheese! Peppermint cream and aloe vera gel are both very cooling and soothing for irritated skin too.*

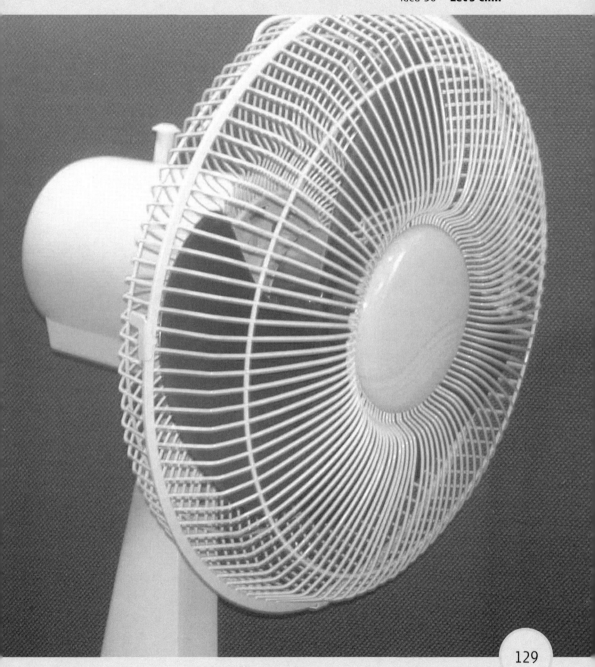

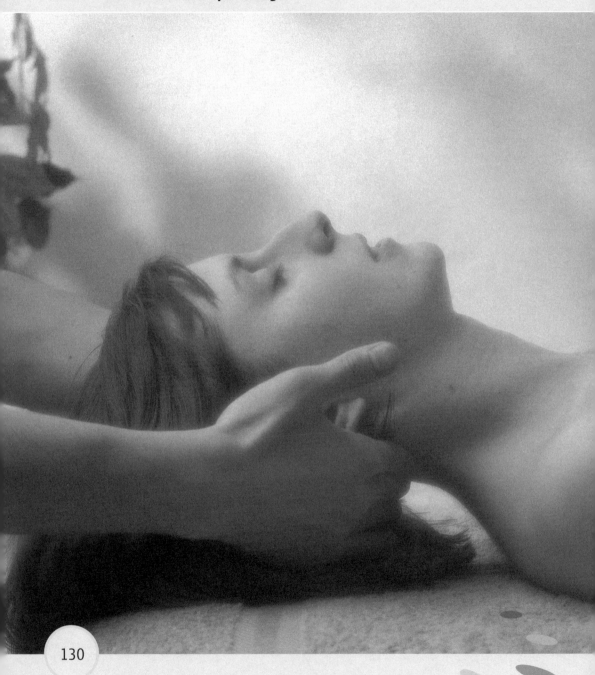

31

De-stress de stress

Stress is all around upsetting the perfect balance of your life. It can set off your allergies, so sit back and relax, and make things easy with a little help from your friends.

It makes us tense and irritable, and generally makes life difficult. It doesn't help allergies either. Keep it in control, however, and the future's clear and bright.

Stress is a fact of life, and there's plenty of it about. We get stressed when we're stuck in traffic congestion, when the post is mostly bills and when, after a hard day's work, the TV goes on the blink or the kids won't go to sleep. Ask most people what they think about stress and they'll say that it's bad for us.

It's true that long-term stress that remains unchecked, that isn't released, is bad for the mind and the body. It contributes to many different health problems – stomach ulcers, irritable bowel syndrome, anxiety and depression being some of the common ones. It can trigger an asthma attack or an eczema flare-up. Basically, bad stress can make allergies worse, which is why it's important to learn how to control and avoid it.

Here's an idea for you... **On a piece of paper write down the days of the week. Next to each day write down one thing that makes you feel relaxed. Now put this list on your fridge door. Over the next week each day do the relaxing thing that you've written there. By doing this you'll make taking time to unwind and look after yourself part of your daily routine and will be helping to control your allergies.**

But let's give stress, like peace, a chance, because not all stress is bad. Believe me, we need some stress in our lives – the good stress, that is. It's what keeps us on our toes and what quickens our reaction times. It's what helps us run away from the mugger or out of the way of the speeding car. It's why we get those feelings before interviews, public speaking and first dates. You know the feeling – when your body wants to be in the toilet rather than on the stage, you can't sit still, and when the moment finally arrives your mouth is dry like sandpaper. Yes, we've all been there. Well this is the effect of stress hormones: adrenaline, which gets the body charged up and ready for action, and endorphins, the body's own natural painkilling chemicals, which improve concentration and quick thinking in a crisis.

So how do you keep your stress under control? Well, the basics are these. Eat a healthy diet, exercise regularly, drink enough non-alcoholic liquid and only safe-recommended amounts of alcohol each day, and get enough sleep. In addition to these foundation principles, take time out every day to relax and unwind in whatever way does it for you! It may be yoga, deep breathing exercises, listening to music, for example. These can be done easily and only take a few minutes. You may want to go to the gym, meet with friends, watch a movie, thrash around a racetrack in a rally car, drive 4x4s through streams and up and down steep inclines, or fire paint-balls at each other. It doesn't matter what you do so long as it helps you to relax. Meditation, for example, is a great way to relax and unwind. The basics involve simply sitting down, closing your eyes, and letting your mind and body unwind and recharge.

Now you know how to avoid stress but occasionally a naughty little stress will slip through. Have a look at IDEA 50, *Occupations dangereux*, to see how to discipline it.

Try another idea...

If you've ever attended an evening class, I expect that it provided you with quality time that you used to relax and enjoy yourself away from the rigours of life. It also gave you the chance to meet new people and develop your skills. This time, being ring-fenced to do something you enjoyed, would have been very relaxing, and it would also have given you something to look forward to.

Feeling relaxed, confident and in control helps to put all of life's problems into perspective and enables us to take on the challenge they bring more effectively. By reducing and hopefully avoiding stress, a trigger for many allergy symptoms, you should be able to lessen the severity of your symptoms, keep them under control and possibly eradicate them entirely. Think of it this way: if it's traffic that's sends you into a jam, you avoid it by trying another route or using a different mode of transport. If being stressed sets off your allergy symptoms, you should try to avoid that too. Simple? Maybe. Highly effective? Definitely.

'Always turn a negative situation into a positive situation.'
MICHAEL JORDAN

Defining idea...

How did it go?

Q   I know yoga helps to control stress. Can it help to control allergies?

A   *Breathing exercises and simple yoga postures can relax the chest muscles and open the airways, improving respiration. Some research has shown that yoga can help to drain mucus from the lungs and help to reduce allergic reactions. If you haven't yet tried yoga, then it would be worth attending a course where a qualified yoga teacher will instruct you. In the meantime, you can try a simple exercise: sit comfortably on the floor with your legs straight out in front of you, raise your arms above your head, stretch toward the ceiling and inhale. Next, reaching for your toes, bend forward and exhale, keeping your back straight. Hold this position for 5–10 seconds, then release. Repeat the exercise three times.*

Q   I'm too busy. I don't have time to relax. What should I do?

A   *If your child or a friend needed you to drop everything and help them, you'd find the time, wouldn't you? So why is it any different for you to find the time for yourself? All you need is to spend 5 minutes twice a day doing something that you find relaxing, whether that be reading, listening to music, surfing the internet or chatting on the phone to a friend. If you really don't think you can manage it, then start off with taking just 5 minutes once a day and build up from there.*

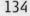

32

Ooh, that feels good!

The sense of touch is a wonderful thing. Comforting, reassuring, arousing – but there's a time and place for everything. It can also help with allergy symptoms too.

Touching conveys many different messages. A hand placed on the shoulder says everything will be all right, arms flung around someone's body say 'I love you'.

Forceful contact through the medium of the clenched fist certainly gets a message across loud and clear. For those with allergies to particular substances or chemicals, then even the slightest contact can do them serious harm. A relaxing massage, however, can have just the opposite effect.

If you've had a massage, then you'll know just how good it can feel – even the most vigorous are eventually deeply satisfying, unless your therapist is overenthusiastic and accidentally debones you in the tenderising process.

A good massage is very, very, and sometimes very, relaxing. In fact, a number of studies have shown that massage therapy can significantly decrease physical and

Here's an idea for you...

Book yourself in for a simple massage. Ask the therapist for an information leaflet about what sorts of massage are available – aromatherapy, sports, for example – so you can decide which one you would prefer. Asking questions beforehand means that you will be more relaxed when you go. And don't be embarrassed, the therapist will have been asked the same thing hundreds of times before.

mental stress. By doing this it can help you and your body deal with your allergies. Lower stress levels reduce the production of histamine and enable your immune system to function better. Bearing in mind that the smell of some strongly scented oils can trigger asthma attacks and that some oils can irritate the skin of those with eczema, it's useful to rub in a small amount as a test patch before your whole body gets covered with it.

If you've not yet experienced the pleasure, and sometimes pain, of a good massage, then you may be a little anxious. That's understandable. You've not had one before, so it's very likely that your understanding of the whole process is based largely on urban myth rather than fact. Locker room or ladies' room talk usually revolves around *Baywatch*-esque therapists who will go to any length to satisfy your wildest dreams. Plus, of course, it depends which country you are in. Just as different countries have different cultural behaviours, so they also have different expectations and techniques when practising massage. When it comes down to the nitty-gritty though, once the excitement of these fantasies has passed and someone has decided to give it a go, the question that is at the forefront of their mind is not how much will it cost and what do I get for that, but how much clothing do I need to remove?

This is why, as with most things in life, a little bit of research and planning is not such a bad idea. I know someone who had never had a massage before. He believed that it wasn't for guys. Anyway, he was much too macho for all that touchy-feely kind of stuff. Many people enthusiastically encouraged him to try one and so, gathering his courage, he made the reservation. The relief to learn that he would be given his treatment with 'Nic' was enormous. After all, if he was going to have a massage, he was going to have a female therapist; no guy was going to rub his hands all over him.

Now you're feeling nice and relaxed you should be in the mood for IDEA 36, *Take a break.*

Try another idea...

Another fear that men have is what happens if you get inadvertently aroused? And this was certainly a concern that my friend had, but hey he thought, she's bound to be impressed. It's fair to say that he was pretty stressed when he went in, not only because of work pressures, which was why he was having the massage in the first place, but because for him it was a step into the unknown. When he came out, the effects were amazing. He appeared to float from the room looking years younger, a dreamy look on his face, followed by 'Nick', the male therapist who had apparently reassured him that if IT did happen, then it would be because he was relaxed, not because his sexual preferences were changing!

Oh, I almost forgot to tell you. My friend suffers with rhinitis, and also reported that his nose, like his head, had never felt so clear.

'How beautiful it is to do nothing, and then rest afterward.'
SPANISH PROVERB

Defining idea...

How did
it go?

Q I'd be embarrassed to be seen naked by other people. Do I have to strip?

A *You don't have to be naked. How much clothing you remove is up to you, and you'll be given a towel to cover your bits anyway. Wear thin cotton clothing if you like. Alternatively, ask a friend or your partner to give you a gentle massage at home. If you know someone who is actually trained to practise massage, so much the better.*

Q I'm not keen on having people touch my skin. Are there any less intimate alternatives?

A *One option is cranial massage. Only your head will be touched, and it can help to relieve the symptoms of allergy, for example, by opening up nasal passages and promoting mucus drainage. Many home massage kits can make massage fun too. Try using a wooden massage roller, for example. Camomile or melissa oil are often used in relaxing massage lotions and can help clean out allergy-related toxins. Alternatively, have a warm bath with some relaxing oils such as lavender.*

Q How can massage help to clear the mucus from your nose and throat?

A *Try this idea. While you lie flat on your back on a surface like a table where your head can be lower than your feet, ask a friend or family member to gently tap the area above the chest, which loosens phlegm, and follow with long, gentle strokes away from your chest and toward your throat to move the phlegm out. If you find that lying down makes your symptoms worse, then try sitting up straight and leaning forwards a little to allow your nasal passages to drain.*

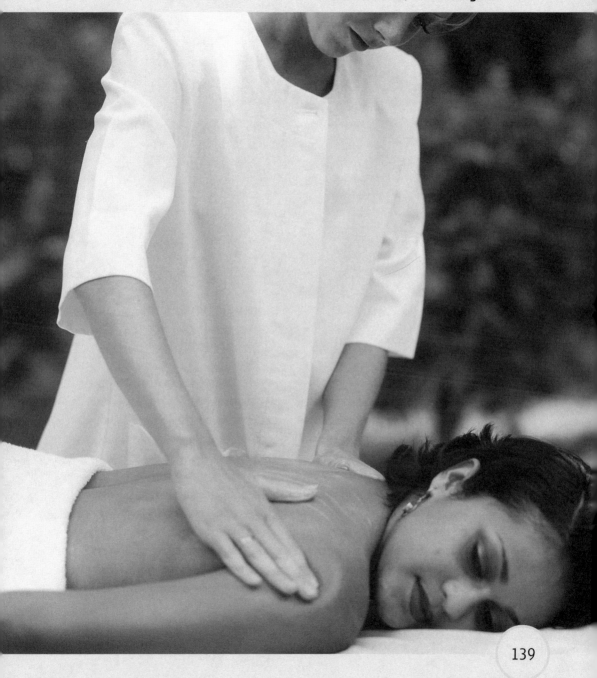

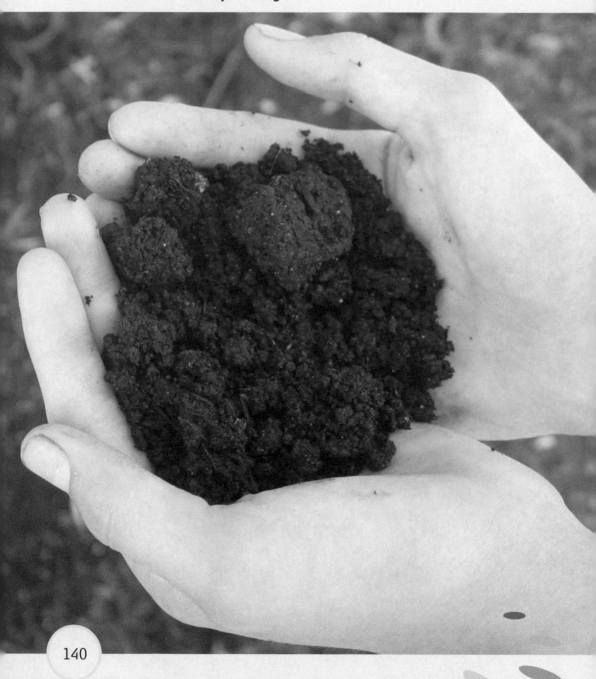

33

A handful of dirt

Dirt never did anyone any harm (live burial notwithstanding), and in fact can be good for you. You wouldn't think that the garden is the best place for you and your allergy, but it may be just what you need.

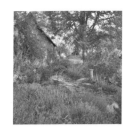

Permission to get dirty, sir? Permission granted. But we're not talking special phone numbers or websites here, we're talking about common or garden everyday dirt.

It's a fact of life that when children play they get messy. That puddle is to jump in, some food should go on my face and onto the floor, this wet mud makes rather cost-effective Play-Doh, don't you think mum? It's how they learn. Adults, on the other hand, like things clean, well most people do. In fact, the increasing number of personal, household and even garden hygiene products now available confirms that we have become cleanliness obsessed. Just look at the hermetically sealed boxes the style gurus are promoting in home-style magazines. Nah. It doesn't work. The pristine white sofa may look fabulous 'dahling', but to keep it this way you certainly don't sit on it, lie on it, or do whatever else you do on a sofa. Well, not after you've

Here's an idea for you...

When you need to clean something up off the floor or to clean a household surface, don't go overboard. Just use a damp cloth and keep the household cleaning products for the special things in life. There's no need to have a sterile environment, which is impossible to achieve anyway. With this idea you'll save yourself time, energy, and some money too.

taken the plastic cover off it. It's crazy, isn't it? I have actually seen a table lamp in someone's home with the plastic still on the shade, and it was all I could do to prevent myself from ripping it off. It's almost as bad as taking perfectly good household items such as lamps and picture frames and covering them in seashells. Though no one would really do that, would they?

At the moment the adults are winning, and cleanliness, if not next to godliness, is at least next door in the dining room. But if we want to win the war on allergies, we may just have to spend a little less time spraying, wiping and washing everything in sight.

For some time now experts in the field of allergy have come to believe that something called the 'hygiene hypothesis' may help to explain the meteoric rise in the number of people with allergies. It goes something like this. If our immune system is exposed to harmless bacteria and viruses early in life, one type of cell in our immune system, the Th1 cells, takes control and trains the body to recognise which foreign invaders pose a threat and which don't. The immune system thus develops normally. If, however, our immune system is not presented with this opportunity to learn, then other immune cells, the Th2 cells, are stimulated. This is bad news, as they try to take control and allergy develops.

Siblings, day care, farms and animals are all good for us, since these may provide the exposure to harmless bugs needed to reduce the risk of allergy developing. Research has found that children who wash their hands more than five times a day and who have two baths a day are more likely to get asthma than those who wash and bath less frequently than this. Other research has identified that teenagers who grew up on farms and were exposed to animals were much less likely to develop asthma than those who did not. Also, children with older brothers or sisters are less likely to develop allergies than only children or first-borns. Now this may not be the whole story, but research like this suggests that being a little grubby is no bad thing.

Now you have got the hang of why a little dirt may be good for you, have a taste of IDEA 12, *Keep it local*, to see how enjoying local produce can help too.

Try another idea...

Not long ago I saw a television advert for a household cleaner which proclaimed how certain items of furniture, for example tabletops, can be heavily laden with bacteria, even more than the toilet itself. Shock horror! It implied that allowing your child or baby to be exposed to these was tantamount to abuse. But most of these bacteria are harmless, and coming into contact with them is unlikely to cause your child harm; on the contrary, it may do her some good by helping to train her immune system to learn that these bacteria are OK, they're harmless. The bottom line is that the hygiene hypothesis says we have become too clean, and in doing this we have allowed allergy to take over.

'In order for something to become clean, something else must become dirty.'
IMBESI's Conservation of Filth Law

Defining idea...

Q   So I don't need to wash then?

A   *Sure, if you want friends to stop calling and people to move away from you on the bus. The theory behind the hygiene hypothesis is not that we shouldn't wash, but that we shouldn't overdo it. There's no need for a sterile environment. Anyway, if you remove harmless bacteria, you provide an opportunity for the dangerous stuff to move in.*

Q   But it's not all down to hygiene, is it?

A   *It's true that the hygiene hypothesis is only one part of the answer, an answer that is still far from complete. In fact, it's only a theory and not a proven fact. Genetics, environment, development and how much allergen a person is exposed to probably all play their part too. Development of allergies is not a simple process and we are still some way from fully understanding it.*

Q   At what stage in life can this hygiene thing have any influence?

A   *It's believed that the battle for control between the Th1 and Th2 cells isn't settled until children are in their first years at school. In fact, this battle may continue right through to adolescence, when another inter-body battle starts – the battle of the puberty hormones. So, based on this, there is still a chance of influencing the process of whether allergy occurs right up until the teenage years. By adulthood it's probably too late, but who knows, in future we may find that even as late on as this there may still be a chance of influencing the development of allergies.*

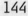

34

Picture this

A brief look at a family photo brings a smile to your face. The thought of a delicious cream cake starts your juices flowing. Have a look at what visualisation can do for your allergies.

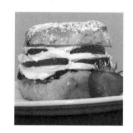

Every day we are surrounded by new images that often just flash before our eyes. Those thoughts stored within the hard-drive of our brain are waiting for you boot them up and run them.

If you've ever imagined being at the beach when trying to relax then you've practised visualisation, which uses the mind to concentrate on visual images. Your thoughts can trigger physical reactions in your body so thinking about the beach relaxes you, unless you've got a particularly strong *Baywatch* obsession. You can use visualisation to achieve your goals whatever they may be, whether it's is winning a gold medal at the Olympics or treating health problems. It can also help you to keep control of your allergies.

Here's an idea for you...

To get the best from this exercise you need to be relaxed. Now picture yourself in a scenario that would normally cause your allergies to flare up – for example, next to your friend's cat. Next, imagine yourself stroking the cat, breathing fully and deeply through your nose without restriction. Doing this will show you how it's possible to overcome your allergy symptoms.

Your thoughts can influence how your body reacts because we all have a mind–body connection centre in the section of the brain that controls automatic processes such as blood pressure, breathing and heart rate. This centre, called the hypothalamus, regulates the part of the nervous system that responds to stress and gets the heart pumping, and the part that calms things down. It's like your foot controlling the accelerator and brake pedals in a car.

If you want to try visualisation for yourself it's quite straightforward. First of all, make sure you are somewhere safe, so not driving your car or sitting on a high stool. Once you're sitting quietly and comfortably, you are ready to begin. With your eyes closed and your stomach soft, start deep breathing in and out and feel the relaxation spread throughout your body.

Are you still with me? Not nodded off yet? Good. Now imagine that your eyes are clear and not itchy, that your nasal passages are clear – that whatever symptom you suffer from has cleared up. This tricks your body into acting that way because, whether the perceptions are real or imagined, your nervous system responds in the same way.

I remember my first visualisation experience. I found myself at a country house on a team-building weekend. It was a Friday, the first of three days of bonding with my colleagues. It wasn't long after we had arrived that I was lying on the floor, eyes closed, surrounded by similarly prone colleagues, being taken on a journey. First we were instructed to find 'our happy place'. Next we were led through some woods. Sunlight filtered through the trees, we felt the cool

The seaside is a great place to visualise. Try IDEA 11, *A dose of sea air*, and experience the benefits of the real thing.

Try another idea...

breeze on our faces and leaves rustling beneath our feet, and we listened to the quiet trickle of water in the stream. It was relaxing, there's no doubt about it. In fact, I'm not a betting man, but I'd wager you are feeling quite relaxed as you read this.

For some it was more relaxing than for others. As I walked through my woods I thought I heard a bear, then some giggling elves. No, I hadn't found some hallucinogenic mushrooms along the route; the person beside me had decided to take a nap in his woods and the snoring had made everyone start laughing. This stressed our leader, who felt we were not taking the journey seriously. He couldn't have been more wrong. The effect on us was quite the opposite. The release of pent-up energy relaxed us so well that the strength of our bonding put us at risk of never leaving that room.

So you can control the uncontrollable. Sounds like something you should have in your box of tricks. Imagine having that sort of power. It brings up images of superheroes, doesn't it? Superman, Spiderman, Batman. Is it an antihistamine? Is it a nasal spray? No, it's Visualisationman! With just the power of his thought he suppresses sneezes, winds up wheezes and sees off sniffs. And you can too.

'I believe in one thing only, the power of the human will.'
JOSEPH STALIN

Defining idea...

How did it go?

Q   I tried and it only helped a little. What could I be doing wrong?

A   *It doesn't always happen easily straight away. Like anything, to get the best out of it you need to practise to sharpen your skill. Try doing it for about 15 minutes twice a day, every day. This way, you'll get into the habit and it'll just happen naturally for you. With practice, anyone can make visualisation work for them. Daydreaming is a good way of getting into the quiet and relaxed state to begin with. Then just let the images from your memory bank of healing visions come into your mind.*

Q   It didn't work for me. Anyway, it sounds like hocus-pocus. Can you persuade me it isn't so?

A   *For any treatment to work you have to believe it can help and be motivated to try it. An open mind is key to using visualisation successfully, which is why children are really good at it. Let's say you have hayfever. All you have to do to get started is close your eyes. Then picture yourself cleaning your nose and eyes with a vacuum cleaner. Next picture yourself without any symptoms, and remember how this feels. Try this for just 5–10 minutes in the morning and the evening every day. Remember, belief can bring relief.*

Q   What about imagery? How does this work?

A   *Visualisation uses the mind to concentrate on visual images, whereas imagery makes use of all the different senses. It's like the image from an overhead projector compared with an all-singing, all-dancing multimedia PowerPoint presentation with added smells and touch.*

35

Summertime, and the living is easy

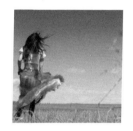

Well it should be, but it isn't always. Clear blue skies, warm sun, traffic congestion, air pollution. Need I say more? With this idea we're bringing the fun back into spring and summer.

It's all very well people telling you to avoid the pollen, but it's everywhere. If you're allergic to it, you can't spend your life hidden away from the world like a hermit.

You can't spend your life in a plastic bubble either. What you need is to take some positive action, and this is why, whether it's hayfever or another allergy that troubles you, a flow chart questionnaire can be very helpful.

Each time you venture outside you take a look at the weather risk factors, don't you? Usually it's just a cursory look to the sky to see whether those clouds look like they're ready to empty, or you lick your finger and hold it in the air to test how cold it feels. You do this because you don't want to get caught out and get soaked, or feel too hot or too cold. Nowadays, of course more accurate weather forecasts are

Create a flow chart questionnaire tailored for your own allergy. If you have perennial rhinitis, include questions such as 'Are windows open for ventilation to reduce house dust mite numbers? Is it time to vacuum the mattress and pillows? Do I have a mask to wear whilst vacuuming?' For eczema, include 'Have I moisturised my skin today? Have I applied my eczema treatment creams? Do I need to get more cream?' In time, running through it will become second nature, but until then keep the flow chart reminder pinned to the fridge or the front door, or both, to improve the chances of your living being easy.

directed at us almost constantly from the radio or TV. Checking the pollen forecast is also a good idea. This will help you to decide whether to leave your home, or to postpone your outing and stay indoors. Of course, if you have hayfever and the pollen forecast is high but you have no choice, then you have to go out, but all is not lost.

All the steps followed to reach a final decision, like those outlined above, can be formalised into a flow chart questionnaire. Answering each question leads you on either to an instruction or another question, depending upon whether you answered 'yes' or 'no'. It's akin to the automated telephone answering services a lot of utilities seem to favour, but less irritating. In fact, I'd wager that these 'if you want to speak to xyz, press 1' services may well be more irritating than pollen for many people as they take you through every numerical combination known to man and around many different countries in the process.

OK, the pollen count is high and you have hayfever. First question. 'Do I have to go outside today?' If the answer is 'no', then this leads you to an instruction to stay indoors, keep the windows closed and return to this question again tomorrow. Whilst you're indoors, prevent stealth pollen entering your home by machine-drying laundry rather than hanging it out to dry, brushing pets before they come back indoors (get someone else to do this if possible), and covering furniture or surfaces that you use regularly with a dust sheet whilst they are not being used and washing the covers at the end of the day.

Now you know how to reduce the risk of allergy attacks in the summer, it's time for you to try IDEA 37, *Let's make a date.*

Try another idea…

If you answered 'yes', then the next question might be 'Do you have to go out at a specific time of the day?' If you answer 'no' to this, then the advice would be to go out after midday, when pollen counts are usually lower. If your answer is yes', then the advice would be to make sure you do the following. Use medication before you leave your home. Keep your car windows closed and, if you have it, use the air-conditioning on recirculate mode. If your car doesn't have air-conditioning, then have a pollen filter fitted. Wear wraparound sunglasses to protect your eyes, and a mask, such as a cycle mask, to prevent pollen getting into your eyes and mouth. If you're not keen on wearing a mask, perhaps because you're a little self-conscious, then smear some Vaseline just inside your nostrils. Oh, and carry any medication you may need with you, and don't forget those tissues. When you return home, strip off in a part of the house that you don't often use, but not somewhere where you have to pass through frequently used parts of the house to get there. Have a shower and wash your hair to get any pollen off your body and out of your hair. Now you know what to do, you're ready to go out and enjoy yourself.

'People rarely succeed unless they have fun in what they are doing.'
DALE CARNEGIE

Defining idea…

151

How did
it go?

Q   I'm allergic to tree pollen – birch, to be precise – but my local weather forecast doesn't mention this. It only talks about grass pollen counts. Where can I get the required information?

A   It's true that, since the majority of people who have hayfever are allergic to grass pollen, it's often only this that is forecast. However, forecasts during the relevant tree pollen seasons are out there – you just have to look around a bit more. Weather forecast sites on the internet will often provide some indication.

Q   Do I need to keep my windows closed at night too?

A   It's a good idea to close your windows at night because after sunset, when the air cools down, pollen which during the day has been lifted high into the atmosphere by warm air falls back to earth. Maybe not with a bump, but with enough energy to get into your body. If you're a hayfever sufferer it will be enough to irritate you, which is why, if you've left the windows open, your lights will be holding back the dark as you desperately search for your hayfever treatments.

Q   Is it a good idea to keep the grass short?

A   As a general rule, mown grass doesn't flower, making it better for those allergic to grass pollen, so cutting your lawn frequently can help. Don't forget to trim the edges too. It's best if someone else cuts the grass for you, but if you must do it yourself then wear a mask and shades, and wash the clothes you've been wearing as soon as possible afterwards.

36

Take a break

A chance to relax and unwind is probably the best medicine. But what if, as you settle back, your peace and tranquillity are disturbed by coughs and sneezes? Good places for a holiday if you're an allergy sufferer.

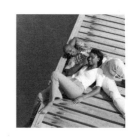

And what about those nasty rashes? No, not those. You've only yourself to blame for that kind of rash. I'm talking about allergic ones, the ones that feel like you've had too much sun when all it's done is rain.

There's no easy answer to the question, 'Where's the best place for a holiday if you have an allergy?' Sorry. If there was, do you think I'd be in my study writing this? No way! I'd be sitting on the veranda of my allergy-free health and relaxation resort writing it, surrounded by piles of cash and hundreds of relaxed, carefree and very grateful people. But don't despair just yet. Even though you may not be able to guarantee an allergy-free vacation, you can still reduce the risk of your allergy spoiling your well-earned break.

Most people focus on their destination when thinking about a holiday. Will it be sunny? What's the food like? Hotel or self-catering? What's the cost? (That last

Here's an idea for you... **Just as you'd research what attractions and tours are available, look into what type of allergy triggers may be lurking at your potential holiday destination. Does the establishment have animals? Is there a vacuum cleaner to vacuum the mattress and pillows before the allergic person sleeps on them? What pollens are commonly around at that time of year? Doing this means you're more likely to have a good break.**

question usually only occurs to the more pragmatic partner, whilst the more flamboyant one is ooh-ing and aah-ing through the glossy brochures or surfing the internet or TV.) Thinking about the finer details is a good idea, though, and is particularly important if you have allergies.

Obviously it's not the best idea to pitch your tent in a field in the height of the summer if you're a hayfever sufferer allergic to grass pollen. I know someone with hayfever who quickly learned that it was a mistake to go on Cub Scout camp, where his days were spent trying to cover his sleeves with triangular outdoor activity achievement badges and his nights were spent trying to tear them off to use as handkerchiefs as he struggled to get to sleep with a nose blocked through inhaling grass pollen.

The desert may not be such a bad choice in that regard, but it's not to everyone's taste. Even if the idea appeals, it's important to be aware that in populated areas trees, shrubs and grasses may have been introduced to make you feel at home. Cruel irony!

How about staying up a mountain? People for many years have gone to 'take the mountain air', often to try and overcome their allergies. Mountainous areas tend to be free of pollution and so make hayfever symptoms less troublesome. They also have less grass pollen, though they can have a fair amount of tree pollen, so hayfever sufferers should learn which pollen sets them off before they set off on vacation. The same goes for forests too, which have an enormous amount of tree pollen. Yes, I know that's obvious, but it's easily overlooked in the romance of the brochure.

Weather can make or break a holiday. It can do the same for allergies. Try IDEA 38, *And now time for the weather*, to see how you can predict whether it's going to do you any favours.

Try another idea...

Traditionally it's to the coast that most people go for their summer holiday. As pollen levels are lower here, it's an appealing option for hayfever sufferers. Though it may not be such a bright idea to rent that rather quaint cottage that's only used once or twice a year, and cleaned less often, if you're sensitive to the house dust mite, since the cottage may be full of these critters just waiting for you to come and feed them. To lessen this risk, make sure the place is cleaned thoroughly before you go, and ask the owners to leave some windows open so that it's ventilated, as this helps keep the house dust mite numbers down. And choosing an educational activity holiday on a farm means those with allergies to animals may spend more time sneezing and scratching than doing anything else.

So the picture is getting clearer. It's about not putting yourself in the firing line or at least, if you really have little choice or say in the matter of where you spend your vacation, taking steps to reduce your exposure to allergy triggers. They say that a change is as good as a rest. Well, play your cards right and your allergy shouldn't cloud your sunny days.

'A vacation is what you take when you can no longer take what you've been taking.'
EARL WILSON, American writer

Defining idea...

How did
it go?

Q I like peace and quiet on my holidays. Could this help with my hayfever?

A   *Yes, it most certainly could! Keeping stress under control helps to keep the symptoms of allergy under control too, so being somewhere that you enjoy is obviously beneficial. In fact, generally speaking, areas populated by humans tend to have grass pollen, as do agricultural areas, so going somewhere away from the madding crowd sounds like just the job. Even though pollen counts in large cities may be lower than in rural areas, pollution can make the symptoms of hayfever feel much worse.*

Q We go on a lot of motoring holidays. My allergies tend to play up whilst we are driving. Any tips?

A   *Just as allergens such as house dust mites and moulds can lurk in the carpeting and upholstery of your home, so can they take up residence in your car. And in the car's ventilation system too. Try this. Before beginning a lengthy trip, open the car windows and run the air-conditioner or heater for at least 10 minutes before you get into the car. Doing this will help remove dust mites and/or moulds that may otherwise upset you. But don't just set your car running, go back into your house and have a nice cup of tea, or the house mites might be gone but the car will be gone too! If it's pollen that sets you off, then a convertible isn't going to be cool for you. It's worth fitting a good pollen filter and keeping the windows closed. If you have air-conditioning, use it – otherwise you'll be liable to overheat.*

37

Let's make a date

Love may be all around on Valentine's Day but that's not all. Your calendar reminds you about important dates, and about your allergies too.

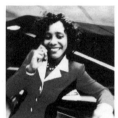

Holidays, anniversaries and birthdays, important dates that without the aid of a reminder would be easy to forget. Doctor appointments, dental appointments and car servicing are the ones that you'd like to forget but dare not.

There are times of the year when allergies are likely to play up. Spring if you're sensitive to tree pollen, summer if it's grass that gets up your nose, and late summer and early autumn if moulds are your poison. Wintertime is when closed windows and central heating make house dust mites more likely to affect those sensitive to its dung, and when cough and cold viruses make asthma attacks more common. Any change in weather conditions can affect those with eczema. And don't forget stressful times of the year, like examinations, when all allergies may be worse.

Here's an idea for you...

Add to your calendar, diary or PDA reminders of when your allergies may strike, when you should start taking your medication and when you might need to visit your doctor for a new prescription. This way you have the best chance of avoiding allergy symptoms altogether.

We can't remember everything all of the time. You go shopping and still forget to buy the most important item. This is why we make lists, and why a calendar reminder is helpful if you have allergies.

Some people know exactly when their allergies are likely to flare up. I know someone who always suffered with hayfever during the last two weeks of June and the first ten days of July. Every year it was the same and in time he learned to get prepared. Why? Because it's a good idea to start taking anti-allergy treatments a few weeks before symptoms are likely to occur. This enables the body to be prepared for the onslaught of pollen or animal dander, or whatever it is that upsets you. Moreover, doing this gives you the best chance of keeping free of symptoms. With hayfever it's relatively easy, since most people have a good idea of when they may be affected. But even so, it's possible to forget what happened last year, and indeed not to even think about it until that irritating itch starts. This is where putting a reminder on a calendar, into your PDA or even onto your computer can help.

But what if your allergies are not seasonal? Well, you can still follow the same principles. When grandma comes to visit, she may not bring her cat because she knows that you are allergic to it. So that's a positive. The problem is, since the saliva-coated hairs are likely to be all over grandma's clothes too, you are still likely to be exposed to them. That's a negative. So what do you do? You can't ban grandma for coming anywhere near you. She won't like that and neither will you. You can't hose her down as she's walking up the front path either. But you can be reminded that she and her furry friend's hair are coming to visit and prepare yourself for the allergenic onslaught.

Paper calendars and diaries are slowly being replaced by electronic equivalents. Peek at IDEA 39, *Welcome to the future*, to see how allergies may be treated in the not too distant future.

Try another idea...

Being reminded about possible forthcoming attractions (maybe *Itchy and Scratchy: The Movie, That Fatal Sneeze* or even *Running Free*, accompanied by some 'eyes scream' perhaps) is a good thing. But having what you need is vital too. So the reminder about your season should also trigger a few routine checks. Do you have all the medicines you need and do you have enough? There's nothing worse than being caught short – in the shower, say, when you reach for the shampoo bottle, give it a hearty squeeze and only a measly dribble comes out. So don't be fooled into thinking that a nasal spray, for example, is ready for action either. And whilst you're checking, confirm that it hasn't passed its use-by date.

Think back to a time when you forgot someone's birthday or a business appointment and thought if only I'd noted this down! If you've ever forgotten your wedding anniversary you'll know exactly how miserable life can suddenly become! With allergies it can be pretty much the same.

'Action is the foundational key to all success.'
PABLO PICASSO

Defining idea...

How did it go?

Q **I hate calendars. I can't stand the way they tie you down. Do I have to use one?**

A *No – your reminders can go anywhere. Leave something lying around that represents your particular allergy, say, a postcard of flowers if you have hayfever, or an empty allergy eye drop bottle, to remind you. Leave it somewhere safe but in plain view, and tell the others in the house not to throw it away. If you put clothes away until the season arrives for them to be worn again, put a reminder in with those clothes worn during your allergy season so that when you take them out you'll be instantly reminded to do the needful.*

Q **I don't know when my allergy season is. How can I find out?**

A *The simplest way is to keep a diary of your symptoms throughout the year. It doesn't have to be complicated. Just record no symptoms, mild symptoms, medium symptoms or severe symptoms each day, noting what and how much medication you needed to take. Over the course of a year you'll be able to pinpoint when the symptoms are likely to occur and prepare for them accordingly. Over a number of years you'll get an even better idea, just like monthly accounts can indicate good and bad financial months.*

Q **I dread looking at my calendar: being reminded of what might be in store just brings me down. What can I do?**

A *You could have a 'good calendar', with reminders for birthdays and days out, and a 'bad calendar' for reminders about less pleasant things, such as your allergies.*

38
And now time for the weather

Pollen counts can be a great help. Find out how to get the best from them and how there's more to the weather forecast than meets the eye.

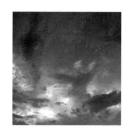

Overnight scattered showers with light winds, and some hail is expected throughout the country. This will be followed by snow tomorrow. So no change there then.

I remember when 'It looks like we're in for a spot of rain' was about as much as we got from a weather forecast. Did it matter? Not really. The adults around me always knew best and often forecasted the weather more accurately – red sky at night, and all that. Now computer-generated visual aids show how and when that band of rain will be upon us and just how hot we can expect it to be. Sadly there's no longer any chance of a stick-on cloud or sun symbol entertaining us by falling off the map behind the weather presenter. All we can hope for now is that the wrong country appears to spoil the presenter's geographical prowess, that one of the attractive female presenters has a Janet Jackson moment, or that one of the male presenters

Here's an idea for you...

Check the pollen count and forecast every day. You can also look on the internet, where some sites will give you the pollen forecast in your area. If you are really interested you may be able to request high pollen count alerts by email or text message. This will enable you to be better prepared for avoiding the pollen and using your treatments.

simply cocks up. For those with allergies, though, the weather and pollen forecast is very helpful.

The pollen count tells you what the count has been over the previous 24-hour period. If you're a hayfever sufferer you probably have a good idea what it was – your sneezing, itchy eyes, nose and throat, and watering nose and eyes would have told you that pollen was out and about. The pollen count forecast is an estimate of how high the pollen count is likely to be on the following day, based on factors such as time of year, recent rainfall, current temperatures and, of course, the weather forecast. And this is of a great deal of use to many people.

If you have hayfever, then it can be controlled in two main ways: by avoiding the pollen and by using medication. The pollen count forecast helps you with both of these. To begin with, it lets someone with hayfever know whether it's worth getting out of bed in the morning, whether it's safe to open the door or windows and, if it is, then what time they should leave and when they need to be safely back indoors again. Pollen count forecasts also let you know whether sunglasses, a cycling mask and some Vaseline smeared just inside each nostril would be helpful, and also whether medication may be necessary.

It's not only the pollen count forecast that provides useful information. Most people, whether they have allergies or not, are interested in whether it is likely to rain or how hot it will be. But this information also helps hayfever sufferers, since pollen counts are much higher on sunny days, especially in the early morning, between 8 and 11 o'clock, and from 5 p.m. onwards as the temperature cools and the pollen falls back down to ground level (the so-called pollen shower). On windy days pollen and mould spores may be blown your way.

Knowing the pollen count means you'll be laughing at your allergies. Try IDEA 40, *You've lost that stuffy feeling*, to see how you can be singing to them too.

Try another idea...

Pollution, the curse of modern city living, also has a part to play in the provision of useful digestible information for hayfever sufferers. Even though pollen counts in large cities may be lower than in rural areas, pollution can make the symptoms of hayfever feel much worse, so knowing how much pollution will be smothering you as you go out and about is also helpful. Pollution level information also helps those with asthma, since symptoms can be worse when levels are high.

Despite being retrospective, the pollen count can be extremely useful by showing not only the day-to-day variations but also when the various seasons start and end, which helps those with hayfever plan how they are going to deal with their season well in advance. All in all, pollen counts and forecasts are something to take note of if you want any chance of being symptom-free.

'Weather forecast for tonight: dark.'
GEORGE CARLIN, comedian, actor and author

Defining idea...

163

Q I suffer with perennial allergic rhinitis because of house dust mite sensitivity so I suffer all year round. Is the weather forecast of any use to me?

A *Yes. Windy days are good days for ventilating and reducing the humidity in your home. This will reduce mite numbers and they'll have less chance to flourish. It's also good weather for drying washed bedding thoroughly outdoors, again so mites have less opportunity to multiply.*

Q My hayfever symptoms appear to have started earlier than usual for the last few years. Is this normal?

A *Climate changes could well be responsible for this. The milder winters experienced in the UK, for example, have encouraged plants to flower and shed their pollen earlier. Milder winters, warmer, wetter springs and warm summers all provide ideal conditions for grass pollen to develop.*

Q How is the pollen count determined?

A *The pollen count is based on the amount of pollen collected at specific sites across the country, either earlier in the day or during the previous day. Despite everything else being hi-tech, pollen counting has remained in the genre of 'traditional is best'. It involves a spore trap on the roof of a building into which air is sucked and where pollen in the air becomes trapped on sticky tape. This is examined under a microscope and the grains of pollen are counted. Et voilà, the number of pollen grains of a certain type per cubic metre of air sampled, averaged over a 24-hour period, gives you the pollen count.*

39

Welcome to the future

They say you can't teach an old dog new tricks. Your body may not be old and your tail is still wagging, so maybe it's not too late for you. Let the class begin.

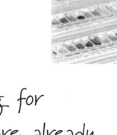

The future of allergy management is already here. Whilst some are preparing for their first-night performance, others are already taking an encore.

Ideas come and ideas go. Some ideas, like computers, cars and the ones in this book (hopefully), become a central and, indeed, an essential part of our lives. Others, like wings worn by men in an attempt to fly like birds, find their place in history. Some ideas, however, are always there in the background waiting for their chance to shine and take centre stage under the spotlight. These ideas are often found in the pages of mail-order catalogues, like implements for removing stones from car tyres, heating devices to warm parts of the body and storage units that incorporate a clock, radio and thermometer, and are waterproof so they can be used in the shower. One treatment for allergies that has had its ups and downs but whose popularity is returning once again is immunotherapy.

Here's an idea for you... **If your allergy symptoms are not being satisfactorily controlled, review what you are doing. Are you practising allergen avoidance well enough? Are you using the medication as directed? Are there other measures you could be taking? If the answers to these questions are Yes, Yes, No, then have a review with your doctor to see if new treatments have become available, or whether immunotherapy is worth considering.**

Immunotherapy has been around for many years. Injections containing increasing amounts of an extract of the allergen that a person is sensitive to are given at regular intervals in an attempt to teach the immune system to live in harmony with the allergen. These injections are usually given weekly during the initial, or build-up, phase, and then once or twice a month during the second, or maintenance, phase. It tends to be used when other treatments have not been successful. Think of it as being like marriage guidance counselling for couples who can't live with each other but can't live without each other either.

For those with hayfever, animal allergy and insect sting allergy, immunotherapy can be very effective. But it does have its risks. Expose someone to something they are allergic to and they are likely to react, sometimes with tragic consequences. This is what happened in the early 1980s, when a number of immunotherapy-related deaths prompted the Committee on Safety of Medicines in the UK to restrict its use. Despite now being widely available and a part of routine allergy treatment in the USA and other developed countries, today in the UK immunotherapy is only now starting to make a reappearance.

If you are going to reap rewards in life you have to take risks. To get the really big money then the risks have to be great too – whether it's investing in the stock market or planning an 'Italian Job'. With allergies it's the same. If you have hayfever and the pollen count is high you have a choice: minimise the risk of symptoms by staying indoors, increase the risk of symptoms by going outside. With immunotherapy the huge reward is fewer symptoms, less need for medication and, most importantly, hayfever sufferers can enjoy the summer, animal lovers can keep their pets and those with insect-sting allergy that triggers severe allergic reactions (anaphylaxis) can live with less risk of death. The downside with immunotherapy is that severe allergic reaction during administration is a possibility – which is why it should only be performed when resuscitation equipment and facilities are available – and, like financial investments or body building, it can take months, often years, to gain the benefits.

You've had a taste of the future; now take a look at IDEA 27, *Sticking the needle in*, to see how the past has now become the present.

Try another idea…

If you're thinking that the solution must be to create something that does the job without the risks then you'd be right. This is already happening as scientists develop substances called allergoids – these are allergens that are modified so that they still teach the immune system to tolerate the target allergen, but don't cause it to react in the process. And what about vaccination? Well, this may not be so far away either. In fact, as we learn more about how and why allergy occurs, the more likely it is that in time it may be preventable in the first place. Then who knows, we may no longer need to go back to the future.

'Vaccination is the medical sacrament corresponding to baptism.'
SAMUEL BUTLER, English author

Defining idea…

How did it go?

Q **It's really difficult to get immunotherapy treatment. Can't I just try a DIY version?**

A *Do not try this at home. Never has this message been quite so important. Immunotherapy carries with it the risk of a life-threatening reaction, so it is essential that it is performed by experts who know what they are doing and can perform life-saving emergency treatment if necessary. Although safety procedures mean that the risk of a bad reaction is greatly minimised nowadays, nothing in life is guaranteed. So no DIY please. It's not easy resuscitating yourself when you're collapsed in a heap on the floor.*

Q **I had immunotherapy for my hayfever because the standard treatments weren't helping. It took a few years, but now I'm able to enjoy summer with my family. Why didn't I do this years ago?**

A *Yours is a very familiar story. For many people, immunotherapy is only used when the usual allergy treatments are just not helping them or because their side effects are actually making their life worse. Invariably it's only used as a final option.*

Q **I'm using the medicines I was prescribed when I first developed my allergy but they don't seem to be working. Is there any point in continuing?**

A *This is actually a common problem, though it shouldn't be. In everyday life, if something doesn't work, you change it or try something different. The same should apply here. There are many different treatments for allergy, so speak to your doctor or pharmacist about a suitable alternative. But first check the use-by date on your medicine, as it may not be helping because it's past it.*

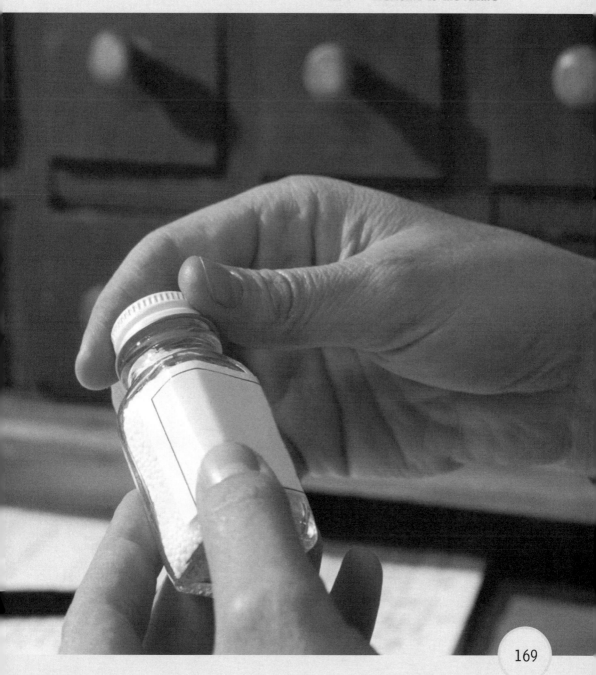

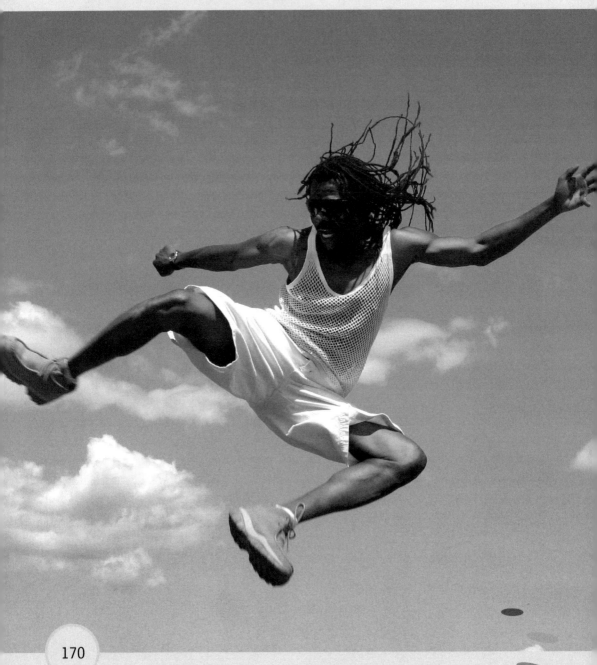

40

You've lost that stuffy feeling

You'll be singing this once you've tried this idea. And you'll be singing it loud and clear too, not like an international tenor wearing a nose clip.

Steam, it conjures up all sorts of images: the early days of train travel, blowing your top in frustration, a hot cup of tea and, of course, energetic passion.

Just as those from the good old US of A expect London to be full of fog, we Brits expect steam to be billowing from every manhole cover in the streets of New York. The thing is, when I was last in New York I did see steam pouring out of those covers. You would have thought that with all that steam entering their airways the New Yorkers' accent wouldn't be quite so nasal! So I'll forgive you if you're feeling a little sceptical about how good steam can be for you, but for those with nasal allergies inhaling steam is just the job.

Congestion in whatever form is a modern-day epidemic. If it's not cars clogging up the roads and adding to our stress levels then it's dust, smoke and other undesirable material stuffing up your nose and sinuses and making your allergy symptoms worse. In spring and summer high levels of pollen make matters worse for hayfever

Here's an idea for you...

Add a few drops of essential oil, such as eucalyptus, olbas or menthol, to a bowl of steaming water. Cover your head with a towel and lower your head over the bowl so that the towel covers the bowl, trapping the steam inside. Don't put your face too close or you'll burn your skin. Close your eyes and breathe slowly and deeply for about 15 minutes.

sufferers; and for sufferers of perennial rhinitis it doesn't matter what time of year it is because they can suffer all year round. The bottom line is that congestion is miserable for both you and those around you. For a start, it affects the way you speak: people can't understand what you're saying, which frustrates both you and the person you are talking to. Being blocked up also makes you feel fed-up and tired, and all you want to do is have a good old pick and pull all that rubbish out. Blow your nose and it isn't any better. In fact, doing this may well make it worse by triggering more congestion-creating mucus to be made.

So what's the alternative? Well, what you can do is take advantage of one of the simplest and most accessible remedies around. You can practise inhaling steam.

As a remedy it's as old as history. Maybe, you remember seeing your grandfather or uncle sitting with his head under a towel, a funny smell in the air around him. When you were young, you may have thought that he was playing hide and seek. When you were a little older you probably thought that he was hiding from grandma's or auntie's wrath, or trying to avoid the washing up. In fact, he was doing none of those things, and nor had your sister draped the towel over his head to stifle the snoring as he slept – you know now that he was inhaling steam laced with congestion-relieving natural oil.

A steam inhalation provides hot, moist air to the respiratory tract. Doing this helps to thin the mucus and relieves congestion. Adding a few drops of eucalyptus oil, for example, which is a volatile oil containing a number of different constituents extracted from the fresh leaves, branch tips and dried leaves of the eucalyptus tree, can be helpful in clearing all kinds of minor health complaints, including congestion, cough, sinusitis and the symptoms of colds and flu.

See how little you need to clear your nose. Try IDEA 41, *Less is more*, to see how homeopathy can help allergies.

Try another idea...

The great advantage of this age-old remedy is that, like all the best health remedies, you can benefit from it pretty much any time, any place, anywhere. It's quick too, needing only around 15 minutes from start to finish. Quick, simple, cheap and effective, what more could you want? It certainly clears nasal passages and sinuses. If only it could do the same for our blocked roads.

'I think of myself as an intelligent, sensitive human being with the soul of a clown which always forces me to blow it at the most important moments.'
JIM MORRISON

Defining idea...

Q I did it once and it made little difference. What am I doing wrong?

A *Steam could be escaping from under the towel, so try using a larger one. Practise the steam inhalation at least twice a day. Up to six times a day is sometimes needed to get any real benefit, especially when someone has a cold or allergy-related congestion.*

How did it go?

Q Is it OK to practise steam inhalation when the nose is not blocked or congested?

A *Yes. In fact, some people practise steam inhalation every day as part of their usual health and hygiene practices, just as they brush their teeth. The scent of eucalyptus is refreshing and some say boosts their strength and energy levels.*

Q I've seen some gadgets for steam inhalation. How do they work?

A *The simplest is a beaker with a fitted cover and a tube. It looks something like a toddler's feeding cup, but with a bigger hole. A moulded mask, which looks like an oxygen mask, is attached to the cover. By putting the mask over the nose and mouth, steam from the beaker can be directly inhaled without it escaping. More hi-tech versions produce a jet of steam, and with these you sit at a safe distance and inhale the steam as it flows into the air.*

Q Any top tips on steam inhalation with oil?

A *Practise often to discover what works best for you, have paper tissues handy to wipe or blow your nose, and when you've finished pour the liquid away down the toilet since as a toilet freshener it's natural and inexpensive!*

41

Less is more

You've already got an allergy, so if someone suggested giving you something that could cause allergy symptoms you'd laugh at them. Well, homeopaths think otherwise.

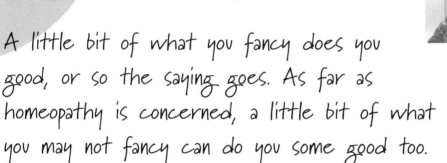

A little bit of what you fancy does you good, or so the saying goes. As far as homeopathy is concerned, a little bit of what you may not fancy can do you some good too.

They had some fun, the health practitioners in days of old. Placing a leech on the body to rid the body of ills, or simply making a hole in the skin and letting blood drain out. Well at the time it was all that was available. Imagine how easy being a doctor would have been. 'Doctor, I have a headache' – 'I'll just relieve you of some blood then'. 'Doctor, I have a skin rash' – 'I have just the treatment for you: take this emetic, and I'll also take some blood from you'. This was the conventional 'scientific' approach, this and barbaric surgery. Imagine, then, the reaction of people when faced with the advice of the founder of homeopathy, the German physician Dr Samuel Hahnemann (1755–1843). The reaction would probably have been the same as it often is nowadays – 'Are you mad? Quick, strap him down and I'll get the leeches', or words to that effect.

Here's an idea for you... **Homeopathic treatments can be either specific or general. Write down a description of your specific allergy symptoms: for example, if you have eczema whether your skin is dry, itchy, burning, red, scaling or weeping, and where on your body it occurs. Then match your symptoms with a suitable homeopathic remedy to try. Consult with your doctor or pharmacist before taking the remedy if you've other health problems or are already taking medication.**

Homeopaths believe that any substance that produces the symptoms of a disease in a healthy person may, in an attenuated form, stimulate recovery in someone suffering from that disease.

Just like his contemporaries, Hahnemann did plenty of experimentation, but at least he had the decency to start on himself first, not some poor sod who had little choice in the matter. He did then experiment on healthy volunteers, although these were probably his family and friends. By doing so he came up with the principles of homeopathy. He discovered that when he took cinchona bark he developed symptoms of malaria. He then used very diluted doses of the same bark to successfully treat people with malaria. From his observations came two principles. 'Like cures like' – the symptoms of an illness were identical to the symptoms experienced by a healthy individual given a drug to treat that illness. And 'less is more', since repeated diluting and succussing (vigorous shaking) a medicine to reduce its potential to poison and cause harm is believed to increase its potential to cure quickly and harmlessly.

Nowadays these principles are used during the preparation of homeopathic remedies. The basic ingredient is dissolved in water, and this solution is diluted over and over again. How dilute is it? Well, think about emptying a can of beer into the sea, or taking a leak in a swimming pool. Ridiculous things to do in reality, I know, but useful for the purpose of analogy.

OK, so many people still believe that homeopaths are taking the swimming pool analogy. After all, if you give something such a good shaking so that it keeps becoming more and more dilute, then surely in time there will be nothing left – or at least, not enough to have an effect? This latter observation is still the most controversial one, but there is plenty of anecdotal and, indeed, some scientific evidence to suggest that homeopathy can help to treat many different health problems. It is widely used in conditions such as irritable bowel syndrome, arthritis, premenstrual syndrome, emotional disorders such as stress and anxiety, and allergies such as asthma, eczema and hayfever.

As with all types of treatment, it is best to consult a qualified expert for advice. In addition to recommending a suitable homeopathic therapy, your homeopath should also be able to provide advice about diet, exercise and lifestyle – the fundamentals of good health. More and more now, homeopathy is being seen as complementary to conventional treatments rather than an alternative since together these two distinctly different approaches can work well. So it's not simply that less is more, it's more that less and more is more – well, more or less.

So less can offer more. Try IDEA 35, *Summertime, and the living is easy*, to see how to get more rather than less from this time of year.

Try another idea...

'*To accomplish great things, we must not only act, but also dream; not only plan, but also believe.*'
ANATOLE FRANCE, author

Defining idea...

How did
it go?

Q **I've been taking my homeopathic remedy for over a month now and haven't noticed any difference in my symptoms. Should I give up?**

A *Homeopathic remedies can take time to work, so be patient. Have a look at the information leaflet to find out how long you should persist. If there is no guidance, then consult your homeopath. It may be that you are using the incorrect potency. As a rough guide, 6c potency is used for most common and long-standing ailments and 30c potency for emergencies and acute symptoms.*

Q **What's the best way of taking homeopathic remedies?**

A *Homeopathic remedies are extremely delicate and so should never be handled directly. Tip the tablets into the cap of the container to avoid touching them with your hands. They should always be taken on a clean palate, so avoid food, drink, smoking and toothpaste for 30 minutes before and after taking the remedy. To preserve their effectiveness keep them in their original container in a dry cupboard away from direct sunlight and, of course, out of the reach of children.*

Q **I tried homeopathy and it made my symptoms worse. Is that supposed to happen?**

A *It's normal for symptoms to get worse before they get better when using homeopathic remedies. Practitioners of homeopathy call this a healing crisis, or aggravation. It's important to be aware of this so you can be prepared and are not surprised when it happens. It's considered a good sign, that the body's natural healing energies have started to counteract the illness. If symptoms persist then you should consult your practitioner.*

42

The mother of all remedies

Handed down from generation to generation, most natural remedies are not new, they're simply making a comeback. Take a look at what Mother Nature has to offer, since mother always knows best.

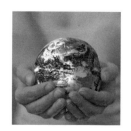

She knows what she's doing, does good old Mother Nature. Why else would she make sure that next to a stinging nettle you'll always find a dock leaf?

Like most people, I've suffered at the hands of stinging nettle hairs as their polished spines injected the irritating chemicals histamine and formic acid. My earliest memories of this are as a child spending holidays with my two aunts in the country. Come to think of it, my first exposure to medicine was probably because of this. One of them rubbed a dock leaf onto the red nettle rash and I watched in amazement as the cool leaf absorbed the pain as its alkali neutralised the acid. (Not that I realised what was happening at the time.) Dock leaves can relieve sunburn too, so can quite literally take the sting out of a crisis. It's a similar principle with wasp stings, where vinegar will neutralise the sting.

Here's an idea for you...

Make yourself a cup of herbal tea, camomile or nettle for example, using dried leaves. Herbal teas are very refreshing, they help to hydrate the body and, with the right herb, can alleviate specific allergy symptoms. But check to ensure it's safe to do so first, particularly if you have an existing medical condition or are taking medication.

Butterbur has been used traditionally as a herbal remedy for seasonal allergies and asthma. Some research has shown that it is as effective, and less sedating, than a commonly prescribed antihistamine for treating hayfever. Other natural antihistamines are the antioxidant quercetin, which can prevent immune system cells from releasing histamine and triggering allergy attacks, and the well-known antioxidant vitamin C, which is believed to also act as an antihistamine.

Itchy, red, runny eyes – now there's attractive, I hear you say. A cold compress soaked in camomile or witch hazel is wonderfully soothing when placed over irritated eyes. As a herbal tea camomile is very relaxing, and soothes a sore, itchy throat. If you can't speak and breathe at the same time, and you certainly can't have a pleasurable snog, then favourites to see you right by relieving stuffy nasal congestion are eucalyptus and thyme. Add the eucalyptus oil to hot water and inhale the steam, and brew the thyme up as a herb tea to drink. Placing menthol, eucalyptus or olbas drops on a handkerchief is a simple and convenient way to get instant relief when you're on a promise, and it will make you smell nice too.

Big red noses may be just what Santa is looking for in his reindeer, but you're probably not so happy with your own. Calendula's your buddy here, and will help to relieve the soreness of that puffy, swollen red nose that is a beacon of troubled times.

With everything in life there's a warning. The value of investments may go down as well as up, it will probably remain sunny but a few scattered showers can't be completely ruled out. If life was risk free it would perfect (dull, but perfect), but the reality is different. It's no different with Mother Nature: just because

Not everyone is as reputable as Mother Nature. Investigate IDEA 47, *That'll be fifty quid, then*, and then you shouldn't find yourself being taken for a ride.

Try another idea...

what she has to offer is natural doesn't mean that it's totally harmless. For example, steam inhalation is great for relieving a stuffy nose, but get too close and you'll get burned, and as well as being painful this is likely to make the nasal swelling worse. Some aromatherapy oils can irritate the skin and their vapours can irritate the lungs. I remember hearing about a flat-dweller who was unfortunate enough to have a leak from the property above. Not just water, but the contents of a toilet that overflowed when flushed. In an attempt to improve the odour she burned some aromatherapy oils. This significantly improved the ambient odour, but triggered a friend's asthma symptoms.

So here's this idea's equivalent to the small type on the label or the Government health warning on the packet: if a remedy is effective enough to do some good, then it's possible that it can

'Nature, time and patience are three great physicians.'
H.G. BOHN, British publisher

Defining idea...

do some harm – by interacting with other therapies or medications, for example. Always consult with your doctor, pharmacist or qualified herbalist before using herbal remedies, particularly if you have other medical conditions or are taking other medication.

These are just a selection of what Mother Nature has to offer, so make use of them. After all, Mother Nature knows best.

How did it go?

Q   How do I make and use a herbal poultice?

A   *A herbal poultice can relieve skin inflammation very effectively. Mash fresh leaves with a little water into a paste and test a little on a small area of skin to make sure that it doesn't cause irritation. Then apply it to your skin, cover with a cloth, and sit back and rest for about 30 minutes before washing it off.*

Q   Can pycnogenol help to control allergies?

A   *Pycnogenol helps because of its anti-inflammatory effects. A natural plant product, it's made from the bark of the European coastal pine and is a very powerful antioxidant. In fact, pycnogenol also activates vitamin C, another antioxidant, and puts it to work.*

Q   What about nettle for allergies? I've heard it can be very good?

A   *Nettle is a natural antihistamine and can help to keep allergy symptoms, particularly irritation and congestion of the nasal passageways, at bay. The sting, which is best avoided, is not present in the cooked or dried plant form. It can be taken as a herbal tea, a root tincture or in capsule form.*

Q   Are Chinese herbs good for treating skin allergies?

A   *Many people benefit from using Chinese herbal remedies, often in herbal tea form. In fact, dramatic results have been achieved. Concerns have been raised, though, since some preparations have been found to contain potentially harmful substances, for example, very potent steroids. For this reason it's important to get a recommendation from your doctor or from a recognised body of Chinese herbal medicine practitioners first.*

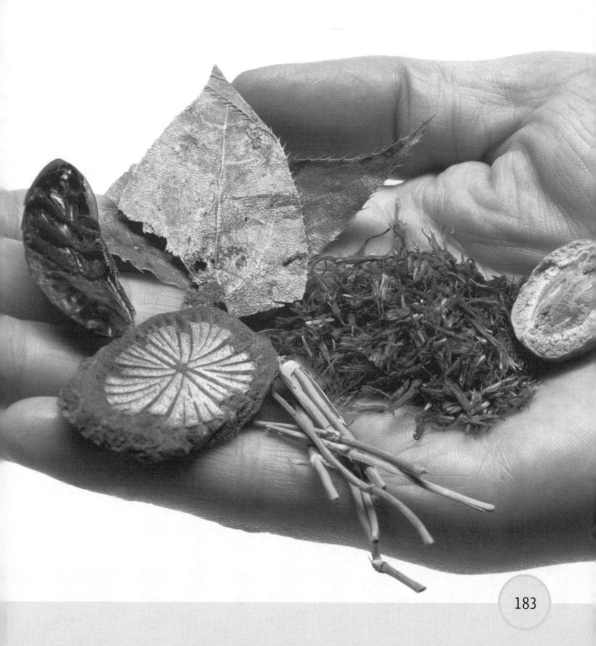

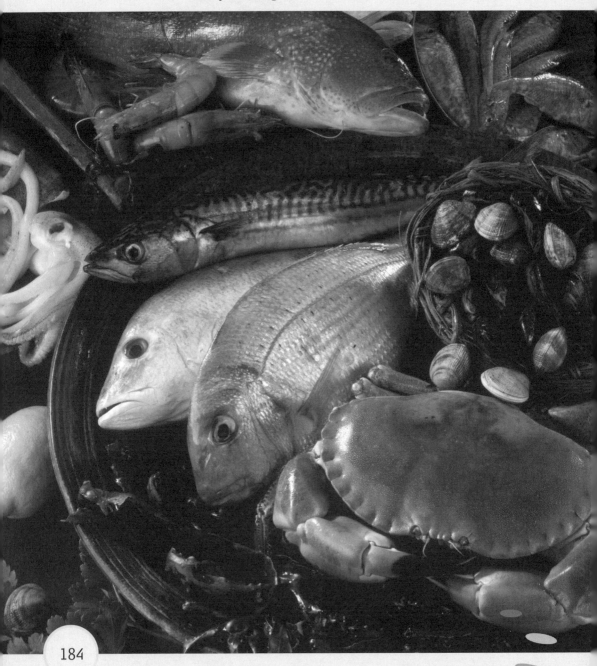

43

Should it stay or should it go?

Excluding food from your diet may help you feel better about yourself, but what should be kept out and what should be allowed in if you're to keep your symptoms at bay? Food elimination made easy.

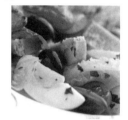

'It's odd doctor, every Friday night I fall down. Doesn't happen any other day. Do you think it could be something that I'm eating?'

If you want to lose weight you need to cut down the fatty, sweet, high calorie stuff. If you want an end to the dry mouth, indigestion, spinning room and woozy-head, then next time you overindulge yourself with alcohol take more water with it. With food intolerance it's not so easy because the symptoms are often quite vague and don't appear immediately after eating the culprit food, so making a cause and effect connection is not so simple, and allergy skin tests won't give you the answer. This is where elimination diets come in.

You want that bloating, diarrhoea, headache, nausea, aching muscles or fatigue to end. And you certainly want to be rid of that persistent feeling of ill-health – you know, the one that's not quite a cold, not quite a tummy upset, not quite a hangover but not quite right either. Elimination is what you need, or rather, you

Here's an idea for you... **If you think that a particular food – bread or chocolate, for example – may be responsible for your symptoms, then try excluding it for a few weeks and see what happens. It's OK to do this on your own, but remember, a more extensive elimination diet than this should only be undertaken with your doctor's approval and ideally under medical supervision.**

need to go through the process of elimination, because elimination diets can help to identify what food or foods may need to be put, at least for the time being, out to pasture.

Here's a red-flag warning. Most experts agree that formal elimination diets should not be commenced unless your doctor has confirmed that it's safe for you to do so. Ideally, elimination diets should be done under medical supervision or under the supervision of someone who is qualified in this area. Not just because, done incorrectly, like any diet, they can lead to problems such as malnutrition, but because it can be hard work and emotionally trying, so having some support can make all the difference.

So how is it done? The process of an elimination diet is broken up into three phases. The first phase is the planning phase, when you decide which foods you usually eat could possibly cause a reaction. These are added to a list, together with any foods that are closely related to them. A separate list is made of foods that are never or hardly ever eaten and can therefore be safely consumed in phase two, the exclusion phase. In this phase, none of the foods included in the first list are eaten. Then it's drum-roll time: does the person become symptom-free? If they do, then not only will they become a new person – they will probably not want to move onto the third stage. This is perfectly understandable as the next stage is the controlled reintroduction of different foods to find out which one will cause their symptoms again. At some stage they are guaranteed to feel worse again, hence the reluctance, but it is important. During this testing, or reintroduction, phase foods are reintroduced one at a time. It's during this time that having a background as a trainspotter is an advantage, as symptoms and exactly what is eaten need to be recorded precisely. In a way, it's similar to pulling a group of suspects off the street. You know one of them is the criminal and whilst he's banged up the streets will be safe, but you don't know which one is actually responsible. In this scenario, you don't let them out one by one and see if another crime takes place, you question them! And that's where the similarity stops. You can't talk to the various food suspects, so you have to reintroduce them into your diet one at a time to see if they trigger symptoms again.

Try IDEA 18, *What's your poison?*, to find out what else might be worth avoiding.

Try another idea...

Elimination diets can be hard work, but the outcome is usually good. If the problematic foods are identified, these can be avoided. If the outcome is that food is not responsible for the symptoms, then this isn't necessarily a bad thing. Other avenues can then be explored to identify what's causing the problem, and at least you'll be able to eat what you like, when you like – within reason, of course, and in moderation.

'To eat is a necessity, but to eat intelligently is an art.'
LA ROCHEFOUCAULD

Defining idea...

Q   How can I begin to identify which foods are causing my symptoms? I eat so many different types!

A   *Part of the planning stage is keeping a detailed food and symptoms diary. This involves recording when your symptoms occur and what you eat and drink throughout the day. Do this for about two weeks to begin with and try to do it during weeks that are 'normal' for you, so not the two weeks you spend on holiday, for example. For some people this is all they need to identify the foods that upset them.*

Q   If I do an elimination diet and identify foods I should avoid, does this mean I can't eat them ever again?

A   *It's a question of pros and cons, and possible risks. You may decide that actually your enjoyment of the problematic food outweighs the upset it causes, and that you can take something for the symptoms anyway. This is often the case with those who suffer with indigestion. They will choose to have their fish and chips knowing that later on they may well need to take medication. Sometimes the sensitivity disappears, so it pays to test the eliminated foods after about a year by reintroducing them. Even if reintroducing the food doesn't cause symptoms, it is wise to avoid returning to previous habits of, say, eating it three times a day. Instead, eat it every three days so that you lessen the chance of your intolerance to it arising again.*

44

'ello Vera

Aloe vera is a wonderful plant that can help our bodies inside and out. Marvellous. What about allergies? Can it help these too? Put the kettle on and let's meet 'our Vera'.

If you're put off by its long, rough, cactus-like characteristics, don't be. Inside it's as soft as a pussycat. But since aloe vera is a member of the lily family that shouldn't come as any surprise.

Originally the aloe plant came from Africa. It has leaves that are long, green and fleshy, and whose edges are lined with spikes. Although it's not clear what specific constituents in aloe are responsible for skin healing, it's believed that substances within it have immune-stimulating, anti-inflammatory and antibacterial actions, and that through these skin healing is promoted. Aloe also has high concentrations of vitamins E and C, zinc and essential fatty acids, all of which are necessary for healthy skin. It's also a very good soothing moisturiser for those people with eczema or other forms of dermatitis. It can help to relieve uncomfortable itching and can also help to keep the skin supple and less likely to become dry and cracked.

It's not easy to get hold of a fresh aloe leaf but it is easy to find aloe gel. Try using some on your skin instead of your usual moisturiser if you have skin allergy, and your doctor or pharmacist confirms that it is OK to do so. It could well help heal the areas of your skin that are irritated.

Many years ago someone I know made a trip to the Caribbean. Whilst strolling along the paradise of a quiet expanse of beautiful white sand enjoying the cool breeze and the palm trees he became aware of a local man approaching him. In this man's arms were green leaves about two feet long. 'You want aloe?' the local person asked. 'No, thank you, I don't smoke', replied my acquaintance, having never seen aloe or marijuana before and assuming it was the latter since he knew it was often offered to tourists. 'Nah man. It's for your skin', laughed the local man. Keen to end this conversation and feeling increasingly anxious, my acquaintance answered, 'I'm sensitive'. The face of the local purveyor of fine things dropped in surprise, and he said sympathetically, 'I'm sorry to hear that man. Respect'. And both continued on their way.

Which was all a little unfortunate for my friend, because what the local man was offering was not the biggest joint you have ever seen but an aloe leaf. The gel inside the leaf can be very soothing for sunburned skin, which my friend clearly had – and was presumably what prompted the 'dealer' to approach him. In fact, aloe gel can be good for helping to treat many different skin problems. As long ago as 1750 BC in Mesopotamia it was used to heal wounds and treat skin infections. The Egyptians and the Greeks used it, and nowadays in modern times it is still used to treat wounds, minor burns and a host of skin irritations. You must have noticed the growing number of commercial skin and even hair-care products that now proudly announce that they contain aloe. For those with skin allergies it's now possible to buy medical examination gloves that are specially treated to remove toxic powders and allergens that cause allergic skin reactions and are coated with aloe vera to act as a soothing moisturiser. This is very helpful when your skin is itchy and all you want to do is tear it to pieces even though in your heart you know this is the last thing you should be doing.

Believe it or not, sneezing is something you can control. Try IDEA 25, *A tissue, a tissue*, to find out how.

Try another idea...

Being alone on that quiet beach with the stranger had made my acquaintance quite uneasy to say the least. Actually, he was what could more accurately be described as 's**t-scared'. The butterflies, the cramping and the urgent need to run to the toilet or behave in an environmentally unfriendly and primitive fashion would have been down to the fight or flight stress reaction. Ironically, if he had calmly accepted the offering and taken some of the aloe orally then it would probably have had a similar effect as, soothing though it may be when applied externally, it's an effective laxative when ingested.

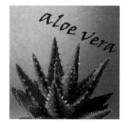

'The art of medicine consists of amusing the patient whilst nature cures the disease.'
VOLTAIRE

Defining idea...

How did
it go?

Q   What about using it with my other creams. Is this OK?

A   *This depends on what other creams that you are using. Many emollient creams contain aloe and can be used all over the skin just as you would use any moisturiser. If you are using a specific aloe gel product then it's best to use it on the areas of your skin that are irritated, using your usual emollient cream as you would normally. If you are using steroid or other medicinal creams or ointments, then it's advisable to check with your doctor or pharmacist beforehand, since it's possible that the aloe gel could interfere with their effectiveness.*

Q   Are some people sensitive to aloe?

A   *Yes, some people are actually sensitive to aloe and it can irritate their skin. Before using any skin cream, ointment or lotion it's important to read the information leaflet and also to do a test patch. Do this by putting a small amount of the product onto the skin – most people choose the inside of their upper arm where if they do develop a problem it's less visible – and wait an hour or two to see if any reaction occurs.*

Q   As it happens, I'm sensitive to aloe. I've heard that honey can be helpful for skin problems. Is this true?

A   *Honey is a very good alternative. It is well known for it's ability to help heal wounds, sores and ulcers – it's amazing how quickly honey can heal leg ulcers that have been resistant to all other treatments. Honey is also believed to have anti-inflammatory actions too. Manuka honey is best known for this purpose.*

45

Send it packing

Smoking doesn't help your health or that of those around you, and you may well find that your allergies are exacerbated by smoking or a smoky environment. So burn your smoking bridges and quit.

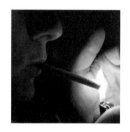

The song tells us 'breaking up is hard to do'. It may as well be 'giving up is hard to do' because it's not easy to give up smoking, kick the habit, ditch the sticks, or whatever you want to call it.

It's true, it's not easy – but it is possible. And anyway, who said that the best achievements in life were easy? When Sir Roger Banister ran a mile in under four minutes, when Neil Armstrong took the first step on the moon or even when David Beckham scored the penalty against Argentina in the 2002 World Cup it took guts and determination. Smoking kills. What's more, it kills people before their time, and it kills those who don't smoke themselves but are around those who do. It can also trigger the symptoms of allergy in those who are allergic, whether they are an active smoker or a passive one.

Here's an idea for you... **Keep the receipts of the packs of cigarettes you've bought. Total them at the end of the week, multiply this by 52, and then write down 10 things that you'd like to have that the amount of money would pay for. This list will provide you with a motivational boost when you're having a hard time staying away from the tobacco shop.**

OK, giving up smoking is not easy. Not for most people anyway. Sure, there are some who just throw the packet of cigarettes in the bin and that's the last time they have physical contact with a cigarette. For most people who decide they want to give up though, it's more of a fag. Nicotine is addictive. Why else would you crave another, and another, burning stick of leaves? Even if you don't smoke, keep reading so you can help your friends.

Many people do not succeed in giving up the first time they try. In fact, most need several strikes before they are out. There are some things, however, that push the odds in your favour. Just like when a hayfever sufferer is going out on a summer's day, the best results come from a little planning and preparation.

First of all, you must have a good reason to want to give up smoking – to improve your health, to have fewer coughs or colds, to reduce the risk of allergies developing, to have fewer allergy symptoms if you are already a sufferer, or to save money. It's like the light bulb joke – how many psychiatrists does it take to change a light bulb? Just one. But the light bulb must want to change. Setting a date is important too. It's probably not a good idea to pick the busiest or most stressful day in your calendar. Choosing a Saturday works for many people if they don't work weekends since it's often a more relaxing day than a workday. And you need rewards to aim for, small things that you can give yourself at the end of each week you have not smoked.

You also need to know how you will beat the craving for a shot of nicotine, which is where nicotine replacement therapy can help. For most people, withdrawal symptoms, which many people are frightened of, usually only last for around four weeks. Smoking is a habit too. How will you occupy your idle hands when the devil is trying to make them work? Puzzles, scribbling on paper, phoning a friend, these are just some of the things that people do to keep their hands from letting them down.

And let's not forget temptation. You need to be ready for when you find yourself in situations where you used to smoke – in the pub or after dinner, for example – all the times when you would normally light up. You know what they say about temptation, it's best to stay clear of it until you can keep it at arm's length. You could, of course, only go to places where smoking is not allowed, this way it's less likely that you will fall victim to temptation. It's not as though you can't go without a cigarette for a period of time; if you've ever been on a long-haul flight where you cannot smoke, you know you can do it. And how many cigarettes do you get through when you're asleep?

After this idea you need a pat on the back, so try IDEA 34, *Picture this.*

Try another idea...

'*Defeat is not the worst of failures. Not to have tried is the true failure.*'
GEORGE E. WOODBERRY, American poetic, critic and teacher

Defining idea...

Here's an idea for you...

Q I don't smoke much, so I wouldn't save much money. What should I use as an incentive?

A   *Fortunately, money isn't everything. Perhaps your health or the health of your children will motivate you. Do you want healthier skin or harder erections? Maybe you'd like more energy, or a better sense of taste and smell. Whatever it is that 'does it' for you, use this as your motivation.*

Q I stop, but within a day or two I'm smoking again. Why can't I keep it up?

A   *You're not doing enough preparation. Write down the reason why you started again and how you will prevent it tripping you up next time, the date you are going to stop, and how you are going to deal with the cravings and temptation to light up. Then give it another go. Preparing and planning greatly increases the chance of successfully giving up.*

Q I tend to smoke when I'm under pressure at work. I'm fine at home. Any tips?

A   *Find a new habit to replace smoking – one that's healthy and you can do in public. Start off with simple stuff, such as running on the spot, eating a piece of fruit, listening to music or performing simple body stretches every time you fancy a cigarette.*

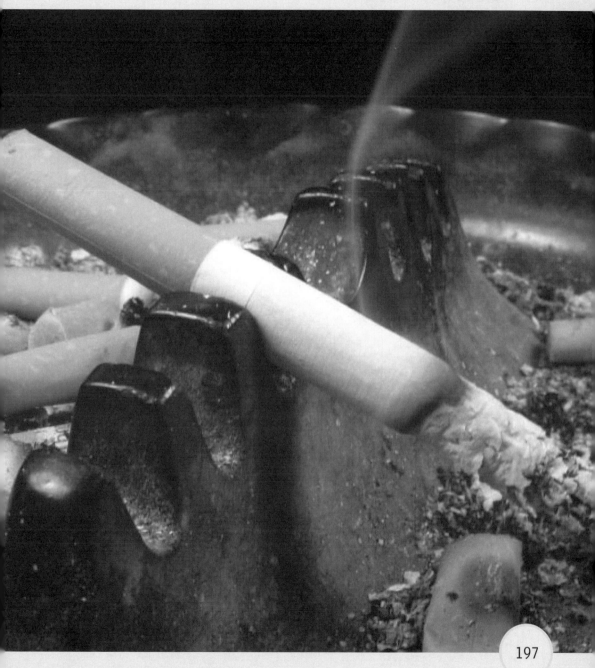

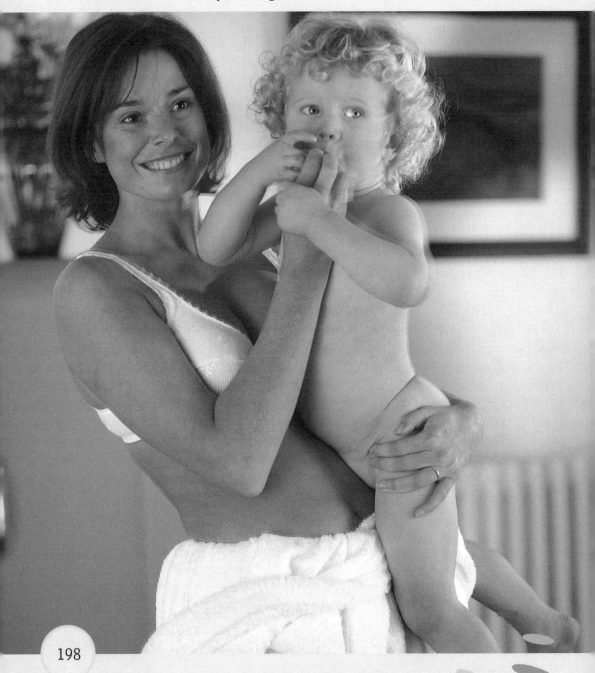

46

Keeping it out of the family

Allergy may be in the genes but it doesn't have to be revealed. Take a look at how to reduce the chances of allergy materialising in your offspring.

We all have the potential to get knocked down by a speeding car, but we take steps to reduce this happening by remembering to stop, look and listen.

Just like the potential to be tall, dark and handsome, whether someone has the capacity to develop allergies depends on their genes. It's inherited. So you may think that there's nothing that can be done to avoid this, but think again. Although you may be born with the genetic capability to become allergic, you will only develop an allergy if you are exposed to allergy-triggering environmental factors. So, despite having the potential to develop allergies, being protected from these environmental factors will reduce the chances of you suffering from them.

OK, let's say the necessary allergy genes are somewhere in your family. Perhaps it's you, one of your children, or someone else in your family who has an allergy. It is

Here's an idea for you...

Make a checklist of the factors that increase your child's risk of developing allergies, whether she already has an allergy or not. Include any symptom triggers for an existing allergy. Over the next week try to eliminate or minimise these. This will reduce the chance of her developing allergies in the first place, and if she already has one it will reduce the chance of her suffering unpleasant allergy attacks and developing more allergies.

possible to reduce the risk of your allergic children developing more allergies (remember that someone with hayfever is more likely to develop asthma and/or eczema, and vice versa), and you can reduce the risk of future offspring being allergic too.

It's time for an analogy, and we're going down the pub for this one. We all have the capacity to get drunk. Whether we get drunk, and how drunk we become, depends upon how much alcohol we can tolerate and how much alcohol our body is exposed to. For instance, I know of someone who's a real cheap date since after two-thirds of a pint of cider he's anybody's. Conversely, there are people who can drink an entire rugby team under the table on a Saturday night and still appear to be sober.

It's similar with allergies. Exposure is a crucial factor, specifically the degree and length of exposure to allergens. Some people who are predisposed to it only need a little exposure for allergy to arise, others need a lot for this to happen. This is why there's hope even when total protection from exposure is obviously impossible – as it is with house dust mite dung and pollen, for example.

To break it down a bit more, things like smoking (during pregnancy or once children are born) and obsessive cleanliness affect the immune system of the allergy-prone so that the person becomes even more likely to become

So now you know what you need to do, pick your way to IDEA 4, *Sticking up your nose.*

Try another idea...

allergic. To continue with the getting drunk analogy, being in the pub plus the added encouragement of your mates means there's more chance of you getting slaughtered than if you were at the vicar's afternoon tea party.

Then there's what and how much allergen – pollen, animal dander and house dust mite dung, for example – you are exposed to because, if you have an allergic tendency, the more exposed you are the more this tendency is likely to become a full-blown allergy. Back to the pub, the more alcohol that gets into your system, the more likely you are to pass out.

It's becoming clearer I hope. So here's what you can do to reduce the chances of allergies developing. Don't smoke whilst pregnant and, once born, protect your child from passive smoking. Breastfeed your child exclusively for at least the first four months and don't wean too early. Keep the amount of house dust mite and its dung down low, and reduce damp too. Remember, a little bit of dirt does a lot of good, so try not to be obsessive about hygiene. Doing these as best you can means there's a good chance that your offspring won't develop allergy or, if they already have an allergy, that they won't develop any more. Then, of course, get yourself down the pub to celebrate!

'*Heredity is nothing but stored environment.*'
LUTHER BURBANK, naturalist

Defining idea...

201

Q **I've heard that having a child at a particular time of the year can increase the risk of them developing hayfever. Is this true?**

A *Allergy-prone babies are most vulnerable to the effects of allergen exposure, for example pollen, during their first year, in particular during the first few months of their life, so being born just before or during the pollen season increases the risk of hayfever. In an ideal world you should try to give birth to your child just after the time that pollen is troublesome in the area where you live, then your baby will be older and therefore less vulnerable when that particular pollen season comes around again. Of course, it isn't always possible to plan a pregnancy so accurately, and even when you do, babies usually decide for themselves when they wish to enter the big wide world!*

Q **I know that breastfeeding provides the best chance of avoiding allergies, but for one reason or another it just didn't happen for me. I'm feeding my baby with formula milk. Is there anything specific I can do?**

A *Many parents feel guilty about not being able to breastfeed, but they shouldn't. Sometimes, no matter how hard you try, it just doesn't happen. It's just a fact of life. It's the same when, despite taking every allergy-reducing measure, a child still develops asthma or eczema. You can only do your best, so don't feel bad. You could try hydrolysates. These are ultra-safe formula feeds derived from cow's milk that have had proteins partially broken down so that the potential for triggering allergy is significantly reduced.*

47

That'll be fifty quid, then

Stand on one leg, hold out your arms and hum. There are better ways of testing for allergies that won't turn your hard-earned cash into a bag full of lotions and potions.

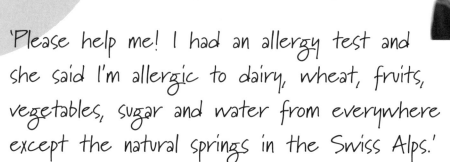

'Please help me! I had an allergy test and she said I'm allergic to dairy, wheat, fruits, vegetables, sugar and water from everywhere except the natural springs in the Swiss Alps.'

So said a patient to a colleague of mine. It's a real story – it's real life. I've seen similar cases, and you may have heard of some too. My colleague's patient was in one heck of a state, and are you surprised? Of course not. She'd been told she was allergic to practically everything and left the allergy testing centre believing that her lunch earlier that day was the last food she would ever eat. But don't worry, she was told, because she could buy all the supplements she would need from Reception on her way out. What she should have done was have a reliable allergy test, but how do you tell which are good and which are bogus?

Many people with allergies are desperately seeking answers and are vulnerable. They're easy prey for those members of society who see an opportunity to make a quick buck. Most experts in the field of allergy agree that there are reliable ways to test for the

Just as you wouldn't buy a car without checking out its service history, certificate of roadworthiness, ownership details and guarantee first, don't have a high-street allergy test without checking the tester's authenticity and insurance. Find out what qualifications they have, whether they are registered with their specialty's regulatory body and whether the test is valid and scientifically proven. Better still, get a recommendation from your doctor.

cause of allergy and there are ways that are no better than deciding an allergy on the roll of a die. If it lands on a six then heaven help you, because it means you're allergic to life.

Skin prick tests do what they say on the packet, and are acknowledged as being reliable. Quick, simple and inexpensive, they are usually the first test recommended when an allergy is suspected as they can test for many different allergens at the same time. Under certain circumstances blood tests may be used to measure the amount of specific antibodies that the immune system has produced to allergens in the blood. This kind of test, called RAST (radioallergosorbent test, as all the boffins out there will know) testing, is useful if rare allergens are suspected, or if pricking allergen into the skin risks anaphylactic reaction. Patch tests are used to identify whether an allergy, and if so, to what, is causing skin irritation or contact dermatitis. Allergens added to Vaseline, for example, are spread onto small metal discs, placed on the skin and stuck down with hypoallergenic sticking tape. About 48 hours later any redness or swelling is noted.

So you see, appropriate tests for allergies have a clear and simple description – skin prick, blood or patch test. It's pretty straightforward and they don't need fancy technical names to prove themselves. Now if anyone tries to blind you with science, or charge you large sums of money whilst trying to sell you the answer to your problems, then beware. Many different scientifically unproven ways are being offered up as allergy tests that conventional medical practitioners don't believe have any role in the diagnosis of true allergy.

Now that you know that forewarned is forearmed, try IDEA 48, Be prepared, so you get the best from your doctor.

Try another idea...

Some of these include: measuring muscle strength or, to give it its awe-inspiring technical name, 'applied kinesiology'; hair analysis, where – yes, you've guessed it– your hair tells you what you are allergic to; leucocytotoxic testing, which involves mixing the patient's white blood cells with an extract of specific food and then measuring the cells in different ways for evidence of some form of change; and of course Vega testing. Widely used in health food stores, a mild electrical voltage is applied with a hand electrode over an acupuncture point on the finger or toe while the patient holds another electrode to complete the circuit. The substance being tested is placed within the electrical circuit and the conductivity across the skin is measured.

The claim to fame of these unproven tests is based on anecdotes, popular mythology and hearsay, which have brought these tests quite a public following. When these, and many other tests like them, have been studied in scientific trials they've been found to have no sound scientific basis, their claims cannot be substantiated and they haven't been able to detect allergies at all.

'Orthodox medicine has not found an answer to your complaint. However, lucky for you, I happen to be a quack.'
RICHTER cartoon caption

Defining idea...

How did it go?

Q **How are skin prick tests done?**

A *A drop of test allergen extract solution is placed on the skin and the skin is pricked through it with the tip of a lancet. If the skin becomes itchy, red and swollen then this is a positive reaction and the person is allergic to the specific allergen. Saline water, which should not cause a reaction, and histamine, which should cause a reaction in everybody, are also pricked into the skin to confirm that the reaction is being caused by the allergen, and not by the sight of the glamorous doctor or nurse!*

Q **I had to stop taking my antihistamines before having my skin tests. Why was this?**

A *Your antihistamines would have made your skin underreactive. Since the test is trying to establish whether you are allergic to specific substances, your antihistamines would have interfered with the test and probably caused an incorrect test result.*

Q **What happens during an applied kinesiology test?**

A *During this scientifically unproven test food samples are either held by the subject or placed under her tongue. The subject then pushes her free arm against the examiner. If the subject finds it difficult to raise her arm, then this purportedly indicates that an allergic response has been detected. Of course, the subject may just be weak or have a bad shoulder.*

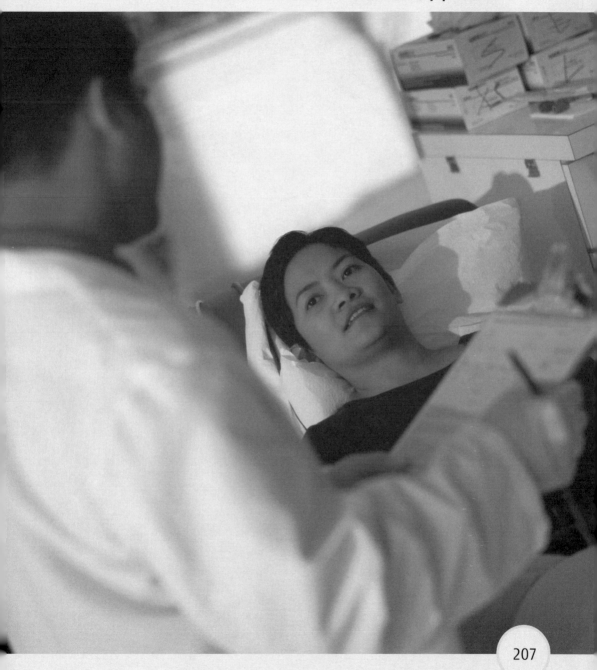

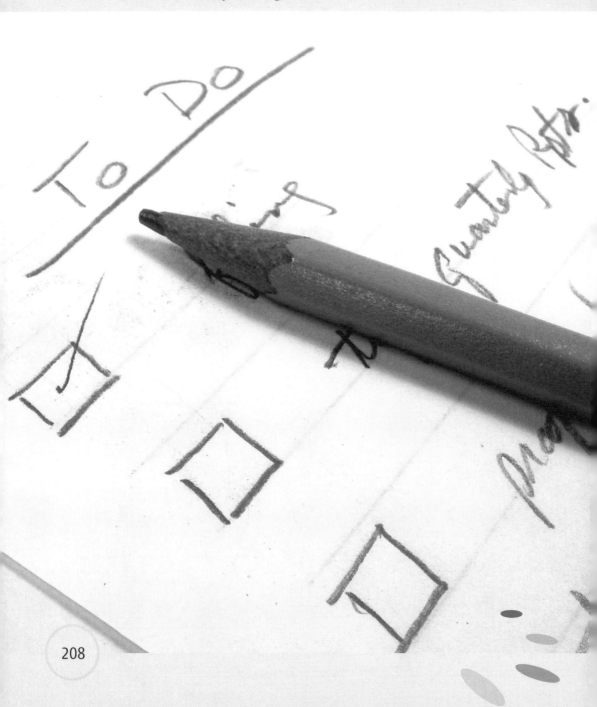

48

Be prepared

Any allergies to medication? A question that doctors love to ask but can you fulfil your side of the bargain? It's time for you to complete the Cub Scout promise.

Preparation is the key, whether you want to give up smoking, plan the perfect dinner or take a holiday. Without good preparation, all you'll have is a recipe for disaster.

Think back to a time when you forgot something. Perhaps you got all the way to the airport only to find that you had forgotten your tickets or your passport. You may have been planning the perfect romantic dinner but, in all the excitement and anticipation, as you strategically placed the candles and inserted your 'seduction' album into the CD player, you forgot to turn the oven on, or to have a supply of condoms available for your 'special' dessert. We've all been there, but fortunately, with the passage of time, episodes like these become an amusing memory, and perhaps a rude reminder not to do that ever again. Where allergies are concerned, however, not being prepared can be far more serious.

Here's an idea for you...

Write down on a piece of paper anything that you're allergic to. Keep it in your wallet or in your handbag, or anywhere where you can find it easily or where someone else can find it if something should happen to you. Better still, keep a few of these pieces of paper in different places, places where you would think to look if you were trying to help someone else.

At the one extreme, if you forget to pack your nasal sprays, eye drops, eczema creams or antihistamine tablets, then you may suffer some irritating congestion, or itchy eyes or skin, but the chances are you'll be able to pop into a pharmacist and get some more. At the other extreme, however, not being prepared can mean the difference between life and death if someone suffers an allergic anaphylactic reaction and doesn't have their adrenaline pen with them.

Doctors do like to ask a lot of questions, and it's not because they don't want their patients to speak freely. It's to try and determine why a person is there, what treatment needs to be given and whether it's safe to give it. A vitally important question that should be asked every time a medicine is prescribed – be it by a doctor, a nurse or even a pharmacist for an over-the-counter medicine – is 'are you allergic to anything?' Specifically the question relates to medicine allergies like penicillin, for instance, which is normally very effective and safe but for a small number of people can cause an unpleasant, and sometimes life-threatening, reaction.

Note, you don't have to wait to be asked. Just tell the person you are consulting what you are allergic to. In fact, tell your friends and work colleagues too. Perhaps posting the information on the side of a bus is a little over the top, but this isn't about being a health whinger, it's about planning and preparation. It's as important as knowing some first aid. It's your insurance, a step you should take so that if something happens you have the best chance of getting through it and successfully coming out the other end.

Imagine doing some DIY; let's say you want to insulate your loft. You don't rush straight to the DIY store and buy rolls of insulation, do you? I hope not. There are at least three important jobs to do first. One is to clear the loft floor, another is to ensure you know how to do the job and the third is to estimate how much material you need. Oh, and if you're a man you'll probably need to go and buy some tools. Men have no control over this compulsion, but hopefully every now and then the tools bought will be appropriate for the job in hand and will get used.

OK, I jest – but the message is clear. Your own preparation and the preparation of those around you are very important if you have allergies; in fact, it's important if you have any medical condition. So go on, get prepared.

Dig into IDEA 33, *A handful of dirt*, to see why advice about allergies is changing.

Try another idea...

'*A man too busy to take care of his health is like a mechanic too busy to take care of his tools.*'
SPANISH PROVERB

Defining idea...

Q   I've put these details in my PDA. What do you think?

A   *If those around you know this, and know how to navigate their way around your PDA, then that's fine. If your PDA is password protected, then it's going to be impossible for someone to access your information without your help, which is not so good. And what would happen if they can't operate your PDA? It's quite common for someone to have a PDA but not be familiar with other types. Some people have difficulty using a TV remote control that isn't their own.*

Q   Is it worth letting other people know about my allergies?

A   *Yes, most definitely. If you are allergic to certain foods, for example, it means they can avoid offering you something that's going to upset you. If you should have a serious allergic reaction, time will be of the essence, and them having the information about your allergy and hopefully knowing what to do is very important.*

Q   If I'm travelling abroad what should I take with me?

A   *It's important to take the treatments you usually need for your allergy. Write their names down and keep this list with important items such as your passport. It's amazing how many people either forget to take their treatments with them, lose them or run out of them when away from home. Also write down on the same piece of paper what it is you are allergic to, and if you're going to a country where you don't speak the language have this translated.*

49

Eat your allergy away

Let's see what's on special offer and what should be in your shopping trolley if you want to eat your allergy symptoms away.

Too much junk food, too much salt, not enough fruit and vegetables. That's the problem. Daily diets are getting worse, the number of people with allergy is on the increase. Coincidence?

An apple a day keeps the doctor away. In fact, an apple, a banana, a glass of 100% fruit juice, a handful of dried apricots and three tablespoons of green peas a day will keep the doctor, nurse and surgeon at arm's length. It will even keep the undertaker away, at least for a while. It may also keep your allergies under control, too.

A poor diet may play some part in the dramatic rise in the number of people suffering with one or more allergies. It doesn't take a MENSA genius to see a possible association here. Over the past 20 years our diets have changed so that in general we eat more processed foods than fresh, more saturated fat and more salt.

Here's an idea for you... **Put pieces of fruit at different places around your home and office, so you can always see them and they're within easy reach. Put some on your desk, by your computer and next to where you sit to watch TV. When you get peckish, eat some. This will help you achieve the recommended five portions of fruit and vegetables a day.**

It's now estimated that around one in four people in the UK will suffer with allergy at some time in their lives, and each year the numbers continue to rise by around 5%.

It's probably not down to diet alone, but there's no harm in adopting a healthy diet that will definitely reduce your risk of developing heart disease, for example, and may well help to prevent you developing allergy or if you already have an allergy to keep it under control. So for starters that means eating the recommended five portions of fruit and vegetables every day.

So what are the power foods that keep allergy at bay? Well, first off is vitamin C, a powerful antioxidant that some research suggests may act as a natural antihistamine. Other antioxidants include vitamin E, which can help prevent asthma developing, selenium, which is really making a name for itself, and good old beta-carotene. Trace elements in food are also important, such as magnesium, believed to keep the airways healthy, and manganese, believed to have anti-allergy properties. Vitamins C and E and beta-carotene also have anti-inflammatory properties that may help decrease the swelling in the airways that causes congestion.

Onions, apples, tea and citrus fruit contain quercetin, a flavonoid that acts as a natural antihistamine by effectively blocking leukotriene and histamine release from mast cells. It's particularly helpful in preventing inflammation in nasal passages.

Make sure you eat some brightly coloured foods, such as tomatoes, and you'll be sure to get lycopenes, another good antioxidant that is also present in tomato products like tomato juice and tomato ketchup.

For good health, food should also be accompanied by exercise, so try IDEA 28, *Activity zone*, to keep the balance right.

Try another idea...

Spicy foods may help so are worth a try. Remember the last time you ate something hot and spicy? It certainly cleared your passages – especially about your nose and sinuses.

And what plays a very important role in life? Water. By hydrating the mucous membranes, water helps clear the airways. The wetter the membrane is, the thinner the mucus becomes and the easier it can drain.

Of course, sadly it's not only about what you eat. It's also about what you eat less of or avoid altogether if you have a proven food allergy. So keep your salt intake low, as not only is this good for blood pressure, it may help to prevent asthma and its symptoms developing too. Some people find that reducing dairy and sugar intake helps to reduce the amount of mucus they produce. And eating foods rich in the omega-3 fatty acids, such as oily fish, can help to relieve the respiratory symptoms of allergy; however, for some people with asthma it may make their symptoms worse, so be aware of this.

It's common sense really, isn't it? To help your allergies, just make sure that the foods in your shopping basket are healthy ones.

'Leave your drugs in the chemist's pot if you can heal the patient with food.'
HIPPOCRATES

Defining idea...

215

How did it go?

Q   Which are the foods with the highest content of antioxidants?

A   *Those fruits and veggies that have rich deep colours are high in natural antioxidants, for example berries, spinach and red grapes. Certain foods are recognised as having a high content of particular antioxidants: for example, citrus fruits are particularly rich in vitamin C. Variety is reputedly the spice of life, so if you find yourself always eating the same old stuff, then challenge yourself to eat a rainbow of fruit and veg every day.*

Q   I've heard that probiotics may be helpful for those with allergies. What are they?

A   *There's been a lot of talk recently about probiotics, the friendly bacteria that our gut needs if it is to function well. On average our gut has around 2 kg of these friendly bugs, which is equivalent to a large bag of sugar. (Now you'll never look at a bag of sugar in the same way again, will you?) Scientific research has shown that taking probiotics in fermented milk or yoghurt drinks, or a probiotic supplement, each day can help to reduce the diarrhoea associated with foreign travel and antibiotic therapy. With regard to allergies, the jury is still out. Some people believe that probiotics may help to keep allergy at bay, and they certainly help to support the immune system, so having a probiotic supplement each day is worth a try.*

50

Occupations dangereux

Plenty of things may be irritating you and your allergies at work. Your boss, the network, and of course the ever-increasing workloads. Here's how to rub out those workplace irritants.

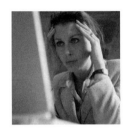

A little stress every now and then does us good. It helps us to perform well and to get ourselves out of tricky situations.

Then there's the bad stress. The continuous, nagging, throbbing pressure that never lets up and makes you want to scream – which is one way of relieving stress but will probably stress those around you, but hey, what comes around goes around. It's important to control stress if you are to keep on top of your allergies. And this is why you need to reach for your instant de-stressors.

Work is one of the most stressful places for anyone to be. Your phone doesn't stop ringing because people keep calling to check you got the email they sent. The photocopier jams, there's no coffee in the kitchen, another reminder email arrives … it doesn't stop. These things are sent to test us, and test us they do. They push our patience to the limit and give us stress we don't need. Like scratching, stress

Here's an idea for you...

The next time your allergy symptoms start to trouble you, reach for your instant de-stressor and use it. You'll find that instead of the stress taking over, and leading you into a rubbing, sneezing or scratching frenzy, you'll be able to relieve the symptoms of your allergy by simply taking control of the situation and being more focused on what you need to do.

can trigger the symptoms of allergies or make them worse. It may be difficult to avoid this kind of stress, but you can deal with it with your immediate de-stressors. Photographs, music, muscle stretching, breathing exercises and poetry are all excellent de-stressors. Laughter is a fabulous de-stressor, which is why automobile organisations suggest laughing out loud rather than shouting or digitally gesticulating out of the window when another driver cuts you up or upsets you, since it lessens the chance of road rage.

Instant de-stressors are simple, quick and practical ways of taking your mind away from the stressful situation. They work by distracting you from your symptoms and from making matters worse – by scratching your nose, your eyes, your skin, even the back of your throat if you suffer with hayfever, for example – since although scratching, and that includes rubbing, initially makes you feel better, it will soon make things worse by triggering the release of histamine, which, amongst other chemicals, starts the cycle again. These instant de-stressors distract you for a moment, allowing you time to gather your thoughts so that you can turn these negative feelings into something positive. They also relax you, which helps ease the symptoms of allergy.

For many people, the touch or smell of a toy reminds them of a happy childhood memory, which distracts them from the problem in hand and instantly makes them feel good. And why do people advise those who are panicking or feeling under pressure to take deep breaths or to have a cup of tea? Because they work. This is why for those with eczema who find themselves stuck in the scratch–itch cycle (no, nothing to do with DJ-ing) distraction management works. It's the same with hayfever: when the brief hit of relief from rubbing the eyes is quickly replaced by more itching, the cycle needs to be broken and that's where distraction can help.

Dealing with stress and playing around can use up a lot of energy. It's time for a short break, so have a look at IDEA 32, *Ooh, that feels good!*

Try another idea…

You're bound to have seen pocket stress books, they work on the same principle. Small and portable, they'd distract you for a few minutes, which is all it takes to gain control of a stressful situation. Executive toys that used to make their home on the desks of directors and CEOs are now marketed as stress management toys for everyone. Their role has not changed. They were always stress managers but it's only recently that it's become acceptable for them to lose their pseudonym. As with increasing levels of stress, so have the number of toys increased. Newton's cradle was one of the earliest examples. Rubber hammers, inflatable punch-bags, twisting cables and puzzles are just some of the others, but the list is endless and there's something to suit everyone. The key is to get used to using the instant de-stressor regularly, and not being afraid to do so because doing this not only controls stress, it helps to control allergy symptoms too.

'Give me a lever long enough and a fulcrum on which to place it, and I shall move the world.'
ARCHIMEDES

Defining idea…

Q   **My colleagues keep playing with my toy and that stresses me out! What should I do?**

A   *Tell them to buy their own! If that doesn't work, keep it hidden – out of sight, out of mind, and all that. Alternatively, leave it there for them to play with and get yourself a new one that's for your eyes only.*

Q   **I work in an open plan office. It's difficult for me use my instant de-stressor – a foam ball I like to throw around the room. What can I do?**

A   *Use a different de-stressor or take a few minutes away from the work area and go somewhere private, such as the coffee area or even the toilet, anywhere you are not likely to disturb others or be disturbed. You could suggest team stress-relieving breaks where you throw the foam ball to each other and so you all benefit. I know of someone who bounces around on a space hopper in and out of the partitioned office space. This relieves his stress and the amusement it brings his colleagues helps them relieve theirs too.*

Q   **My stress toy doesn't appear to be so effective anymore. Should I simply persevere or can I cut it into little bits with my staple remover?**

A   *It sounds as though you are starting to associate your de-stressor with stress, rather than relaxation. In this case it's worth trying something different for a while. Puzzles such as Rubik's cube, computer games and games on mobile phones can have a similar effect. They initially start out by providing a break, which is relaxing. However, since they challenge the user this can create some degree of stress.*

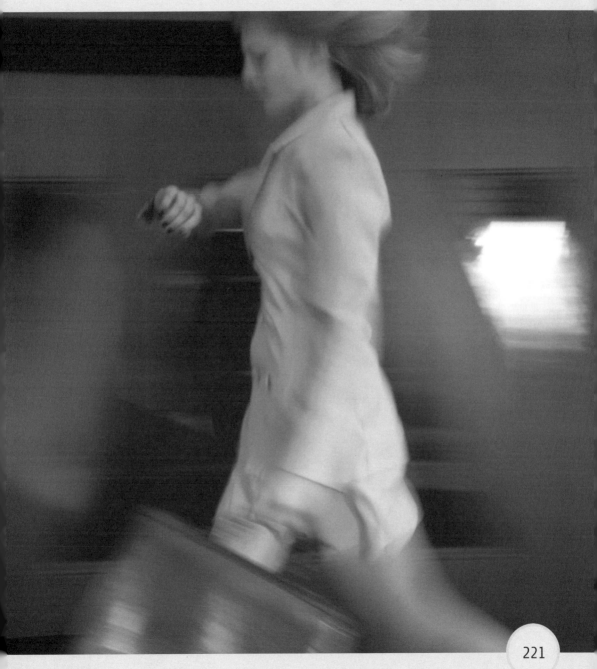

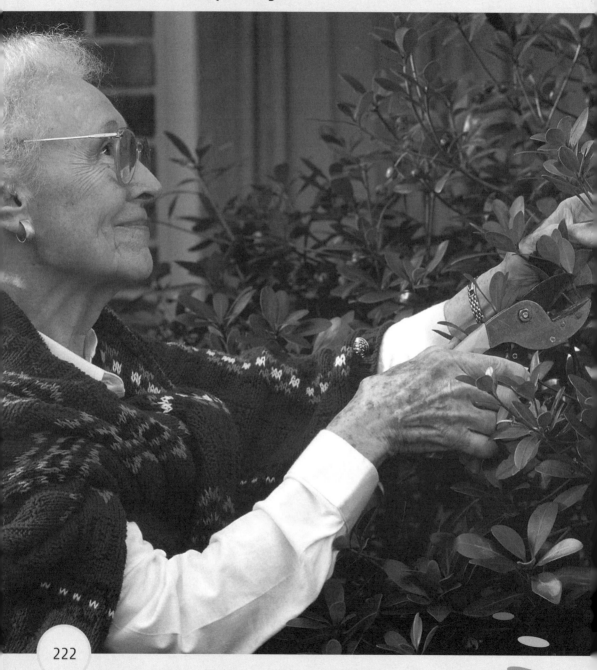

51

Dad's Daily Dose

Everyone has their favourite remedy for treating common ailments. Here are some that have been passed down through my family.

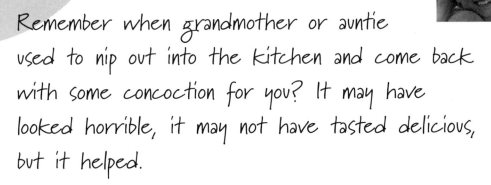

Remember when grandmother or auntie used to nip out into the kitchen and come back with some concoction for you? It may have looked horrible, it may not have tasted delicious, but it helped.

Look back far enough, or ask enough people, and you'll usually find that many, if not most, of the remedies used for allergies today have been around for years. Old wives' tales often make a lot of sense, so it's important not to dismiss them. Likewise, many of the home remedies that have been handed down through the generations do work. For instance, the dock leaf to soothe the sting of a nettle, some honey for an itchy sore throat, and ice for anything that's uncomfortably swollen. They may have gone through a bit of a makeover to bring them up to date and make them 'new and improved', but essentially they're the same. This is why it's important to keep hold of these, just as you would your family's history.

Here's an idea for you...

Talk to older relatives to find out what remedies your family have used through the generations to overcome the symptoms of allergy and how well they worked. Record how to make them and keep them in a ledger so you can pass them on to future generations. By doing this you'll always have them to hand when you need to use them and, you never know, in time they may make your family's fortune.

I'll never forget how excited I was to have discovered the benefits of herbal teas, camomile tea to be precise. I couldn't wait to share my new discovery with my patients. Having found someone for whom I thought it would be of benefit, I smiled and launched into an explanation of why I thought that camomile tea would be just the thing for her problem. 'Yes, I know,' my patient replied, 'we've used that for years in our family.' I was deflated, but there was no need to be because I had reassured my patient and had actually strengthened her trust in me.

It's easy to dismiss folklore like this, but you should try the idea first, before kicking it into touch. 'Verrucas will disappear of their own accord in time but usually it's not easy to speed the process up.' Wrong! Not if you stick the inside of a banana skin or some duct tape to them. Don't believe me? Try it.

But I digress. It's allergies we are discussing here: snotty noses, runny eyes and sneezing to make sure that everyone benefits from your extra mucus production. Lovely.

Let's face it, you may laugh when you think about hiding your head under a towel and leaning over a bowl of hot water, but you're smiling once you've done it and can breathe easily again. Warm water with fresh lemon and a spoonful of honey added to it works wonders for a sore and itchy throat when first gargled and then swallowed.

There's a reason or two to get those shades on in IDEA 5, *It's a wrap*. That's if you need an excuse.

Try another idea...

Growing up, it was always a glass of warm water, a spoonful of honey and a few drops of lemon and vinegar that I was given before going to bed to ease my hayfever symptoms so that through the night I, and the rest of my family, could get some sleep. It was my father who came up with the idea, and so during the hayfever season within our family it became affectionately known as Dad's Daily Dose. It worked, too. On many occasions I have asked whether there wasn't just a hint of whisky or brandy included in it as well. But the response I receive is always the same: 'no son, I don't think so, but then it was some time ago'. Like most home-made family remedies, over time the recipe would have been tweaked now and again. Something new may be added, something else taken out or forgotten. There really is only one way to find out if something works or not, and that's to try it. With home-made remedies that's usually fine, provided it's safe, of course. Ideally test it on yourself before you lay it on anyone else, even if it's been in the family for generations, because every now and then some things are best kept within the family, like the time when ...

'Let food be thy medicine, thy medicine shall be thy food.'
HIPPOCRATES

Defining idea...

How did
it go?

Q Any tips for itchy skin?

A *Combine equal parts of cider vinegar and water. Dab this onto the affected
area and let it dry. You can repeat this as often as needed. Likewise,
calamine lotion can be dabbed on and left to dry. Bicarbonate of soda, or
baking soda, is an old favourite. Add a tablespoon of soda to a cupful of
water and wash the affected area with this solution.*

**Q I have always used fruit smoothies to ease my allergy symptoms.
It's something we have done in our family for years, although it's
much easier now we've invested in a blender! Do they really work
or do they just taste good?**

A *Smoothies are not only delicious in themselves, they are a wonderful way of
providing the body with the vitamins and minerals it needs. In particular,
strawberries, blackcurrants and kiwi fruit contain large amounts of the
antioxidant vitamin C, which, amongst its other health benefits, is believed
to have an antihistamine action. Adding a little honey makes it richly
soothing and will sweeten the smoothie if necessary. Alternatively some
freshly squeezed lemon juice provides extra vitamin C and gives it some
zing. If dairy products make your congestion worse, then try juicing instead.*

Q How can grape seed extract help in allergy treatment?

A *Grape seed extract is believed to act as a natural antihistamine and through
this action can help to lessen allergy symptoms such as sneezing and
congestion. It is thought to also inhibit the release of prostaglandins,
chemicals that can generate inflammation during an allergy attack, and so
reduce the symptoms associated with hives, eczema and hayfever.*

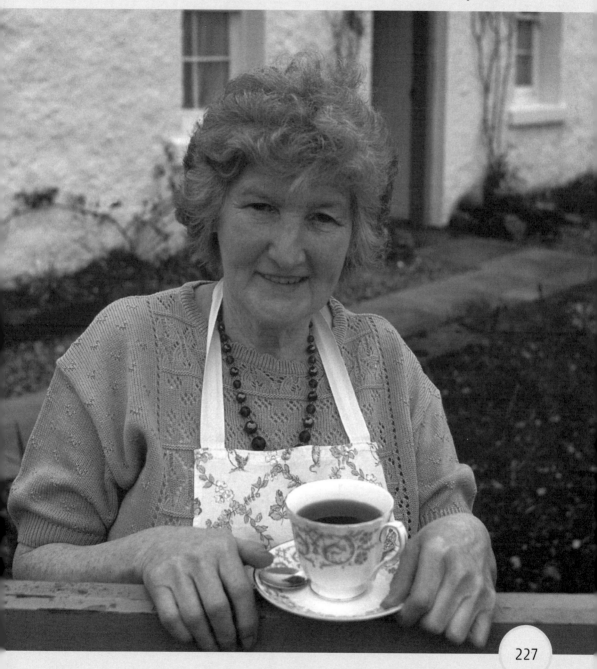

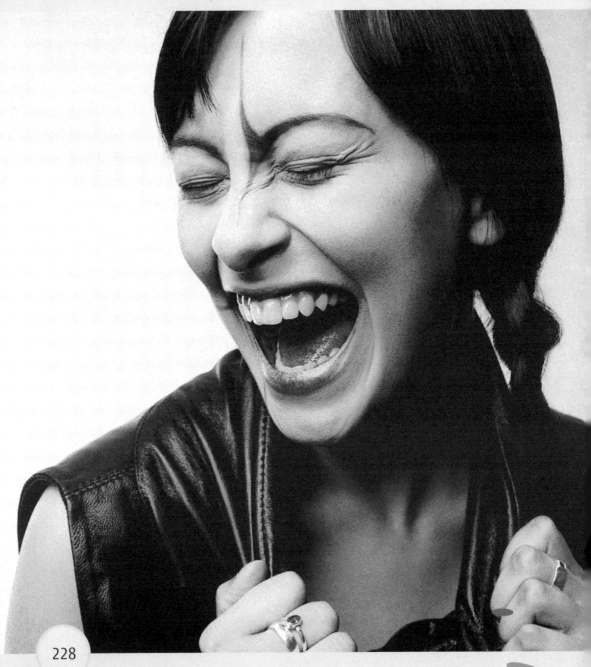

52

Go on, you've earned it

Taking time out to enjoy yourself can help to keep allergy symptoms at bay. Don't be shy, reward yourself. After all, a little bit of what you fancy does you good.

Some of the best things in life may be free, but the things that bring most satisfaction are those we feel we deserve, that we've earned. So go on, it's time to take your reward.

There's often too much health advice that says don't do this, don't do that. Times are changing though, and at last many activities and pleasures we have enjoyed in the past are back on the menu. Something that's never disappeared from it, however, is rewarding yourself.

It makes us feel good to be rewarded for doing something well. For most people with allergies being symptom-free is usually reward enough. But why not double that reward? Not double or nothing, but a guaranteed double reward – no symptoms plus a massage, for example. Sounds good. Interested? Then read on.

Tell someone not to do something and they'll probably go ahead and do it. I remember sitting in a religious education class and the first thing the teacher said

Here's an idea for you...

Write something you have to do on the left-hand side of a sheet of paper – a report, more exercise, for example. Draw an arrow from it to the right hand side of the page. At the head of the arrow write down something you would like as a reward for completing the task. Once the item on the left is actioned, you action the item on the right. By doing this you've made having a reward easy by making it something you must do.

was, 'don't turn around and look at the door'. I'd say that the whole class turned around. So if you're told to reward yourself, based on this principle you probably wouldn't. Not because you are an insolent teenager with hormone issues either, but because as far as you're concerned, to paraphrase *Wayne's World*, you're not worthy.

It's OK if someone else is rewarding you, though. After all, from the onset of our lives we are surrounded with rewards from others. As toddlers, weeing into the potty rather than onto the floor was rewarded with clapping or approval from mummy and daddy. As we grew older, eating our greens and behaving ourselves meant we could stay up late. Pass our exams and the car was ours on the weekend. Once we'd left the security of our family home rewards became promotions, bonuses, a better car, a bigger house. But rewarding yourself, well that can be hard.

The reward system facilitates actions that we are either in the process of learning, like potty training, or that we already know we should be doing but need a little encouragement to do. It's a motivator. Take smoking, for instance. If you smoke you'll be aware that it's bad for your health. As far as your health is concerned, you should stop. Simple. But this may not be reward enough for some. Anyway, we may accept that a reward is on the cards, but when it comes we're not very good at taking that reward and acknowledging that we've done something to deserve it. We often feel guilty about spoiling ourselves and need someone to give us permission, to allow us to take our reward, which is why a lot of health advice has turned around from 'don't' to 'it's OK to …'.

Whilst we're on the subject of celebrating success, try IDEA 49, *Eat your allergy away.*

Try another idea…

One way of overcoming these barriers is to think of something you have to do in the next week or so that will take a bit of effort, that you may find a challenge and that, given the chance, you'd rather not have to do. It may be something work-related, like a presentation, or health-related, like cutting down the amount of salt you have each day. Once you've completed your challenge, go and do something that you enjoy. It doesn't matter what it is, but afterwards you'll realise how good you feel and how easy it was. You see, you're learning to reward yourself and to feel comfortable with this already.

If you have an allergy, let's say hayfever, and you've avoided the pollen the best you can and taken your medicine on time, you will now have hardly any symptoms. Great! Well done! Now reward yourself. No, not having symptoms isn't enough, because this is how it should be for you all the time. You need a reward as … well, as a reward!

'Every day in every way, I am getting better and better.'
EMILE COUE, French psychotherapist

Defining idea…

231

Q   It's taking me ages. I don't feel I'm ever going to reach my reward – can I cheat?

A   *Certainly not! But you have set the target too high. The problem is that you'll give up trying, since your reward isn't even a light at the end of the tunnel yet. Try breaking your task down into smaller, achievable chunks. For example, if you've decided that your reward comes once you've eaten five portions of fruit and vegetables a day for a week, allow yourself a reward once you've done this for 4 days. Then have another reward after 5 days, and so on. This way, not only will you get your rewards – you'll also remain positive and motivated to keep going.*

Q   I always feel self-indulgent when I do things I like. Can you help me?

A   *Let's say you want to have a massage, just because you want one. This probably won't be a good enough reason for you, so you'll need to justify it. What you would normally say is, 'I've worked really hard this week on that report, and after all the hours in front of the computer my neck is really giving me some trouble, so I'll have a massage'. See how you've had to find a negative, the pain in the neck, to justify it. It should be like this – 'I've worked really hard on that report this week. I've met the deadline and my boss is delighted. I'm going to have a massage.' You've done something well, so reward yourself. Of course, it doesn't have to be a massage; your reward can be anything you want.*

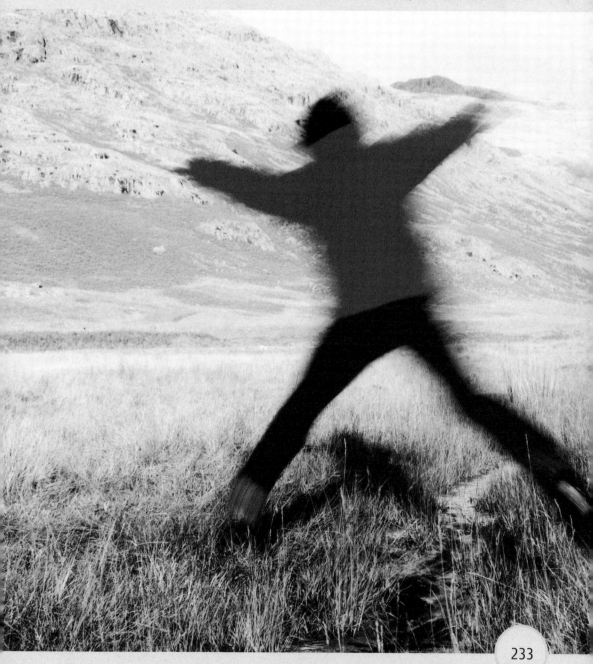

The end...

Or is it a new beginning?

We hope that the ideas in this book will have inspired you to try some new things to combat your wheezes and sneezes. We hope you've found that making small but effective lifestyle changes has worked and that you're already reaching for your shades, vacuuming with glee, taking five minutes to relax and much, much more without even having to think about it. You should be well on your way to a healthier, fitter, more fulfilled and balanced you, brimming with good intentions.

You're mean, you're motivated and you don't care who knows it.

So why not let us know all about it? Tell us how you got on. What did it for you – what helped you to ditch the itch at last? Maybe you've got some tips of your own you want to share (see next page if so). And if you liked this book you may find we have even more brilliant ideas that could change other areas of your life for the better.

You'll find the Infinite Ideas crew waiting for you online at www.infideas.com.

Or if you prefer to write, then send your letters to:
Beat your allergies
The Infinite Ideas Company Ltd
36 St Giles, Oxford OX1 3LD, United Kingdom

We want to know what you think, because we're all working on making our lives better too. Give us your feedback and you could win a copy of another 52 *Brilliant Ideas* book of your choice. Or maybe get a crack at writing your own.

Good luck. Be brilliant.

Offer one

CASH IN YOUR IDEAS

We hope you enjoy this book. We hope it inspires, amuses, educates and entertains you. But we don't assume that you're a novice, or that this is the first book that you've bought on the subject. You've got ideas of your own. Maybe our author has missed an idea that you use successfully. If so, why not send it to info@infideas.com, and if we like it we'll post it on our bulletin board. Better still, if your idea makes it into print we'll send you £50 and you'll be fully credited so that everyone knows you've had another Brilliant Idea.

Offer two

HOW COULD YOU REFUSE?

Amazing discounts on bulk quantities of Infinite Ideas books are available to corporations, professional associations and other organizations.

For details call us on:
+44 (0)1865 514888
fax: +44 (0)1865 514777
or e-mail: info@infideas.com

Where it's at...